NORTH CAROLINA
STATE BOARD OF COMMUNITY COLLEGES
LIBRARIES
SAMPSON COMMUNITY COLLEGE

Divorce and the Next Generation: Effects on Young Adults' Patterns of Intimacy and Expectations for Marriage

ALL HAWORTH BOOKS & JOURNALS
ARE PRINTED ON CERTIFIED
ACID-FREE PAPER

Divorce and the Next Generation: Effects on Young Adults' Patterns of Intimacy and Expectations for Marriage

Craig A. Everett, PhD
Editor

The Haworth Press, Inc.
New York • London • Norwood (Australia)

Divorce and the Next Generation: Effects on Young Adults' Patterns of Intimacy and Expectations for Marriage has also been published as *Journal of Divorce & Remarriage*, Volume 18, Numbers 3/4 1992.

© 1992 by The Haworth Press, Inc. All rights reserved. No part of this work may be reproduced or utilized in any form or by any means, electronic or mechanical, including photocopying, microfilm and recording, or by any information storage and retrieval system, without permission in writing from the publisher. Printed in the United States of America.

The Haworth Press, Inc., 10 Alice Street, Binghamton, NY 13904-1580 USA

Library of Congress Cataloging-in-Publication Data

Divorce and the next generation : effects on young adults' patterns of intimacy and expectations for marriage / Craig A. Everett, editor.
     p. cm.
     "Published as Journal of Divorce & Remarriage, volume 18, numbers 3/4, 1992"-T.P. verso.
     Includes bibliographical references.
     ISBN 1-56024-444-5 (alk. paper)
     1. Adult children of divorced parents–United States–Attitudes. 2. College students–United States–Attitudes. 3. marriage–United States. 4. Intimacy (Psychology) I. Everett, Craig A.
HQ777.5.5D55 1992
306.89–dc20
                                                                         92-43097
                                                                                       CIP

Divorce and the Next Generation: Effects on Young Adults' Patterns of Intimacy and Expectations for Marriage

CONTENTS

ABOUT THE EDITOR

Craig A. Everett, PhD, is a marriage and family therapist in private practice in Tucson, Arizona, and Director of the Arizona Institute of Family Therapy. In addition to his 20 years of experience in clinical practice, he was formerly President of the American Association for Marriage and Family Therapy. Dr. Everett's previous positions include Director of Family Therapy Training and Associate Professor at both Florida State University and Auburn University. He has been the editor of the *Journal of Divorce & Remarriage* (formerly the *Journal of Divorce*) since 1983 and is an editorial board member of six professional journals.

Introduction

Clinicians recognize on an everyday basis that children of divorced families carry with them extra dimensions of developmental struggles into their young adulthood and later into their adult relationships. Even in families where the parent's divorce was amicable, the emerging young adults may approach their formation of relationships with extra neediness, or perhaps greater caution, or even avoidance. All of our own patterns of mate selection and intimacy are shaped, at least in part, by the parental models and experiences in our families of origin. When that experience is disrupted by the hurt and anger of a parental divorce, one can no longer approach intimacy and marriage with the innocence and expectations often idealized in our culture.

This volume attempts to address the complex picture of how the experience of divorce in one generation may influence the next generation's approach to and preparedness for marriage. The only data available to look at these patterns has been the research which compares differing variables of developmental achievement, personal adjustment, and attitudes of children from divorced and nondivorced families.

The studies selected in this work focus primarily on young adults and the patterns and attitudes regarding intimacy and attachment that they will carry into their own adult marriages. Much of the research is limited in that it utilizes convenient populations of college students, so one must be careful generalizing to other groups. However, I believe that the implications of these findings for beginning to understand this intergenerational effect from divorce in one generation to marriage in the next generation are crucial and outweigh the limitations. I know many colleagues would argue against utilizing these studies to form a whole edited volume. However, it is my hope that these works will provide both a foundation and a stimulus for much more extensive research into these dynamics,

© 1992 by The Haworth Press, Inc. All rights reserved.

and that many of the findings reported here will better inform those of us who work with divorcing families and young adults in clinical and educational settings.

Craig A. Everett
Tucson, Arizona

The Effects of Childhood Family Structure and Perceptions of Parents' Marital Happiness on Familial Aspirations

Marion C. Willetts-Bloom
Steven L. Nock

SUMMARY. The effects of parents' marital dissolution and the perceived happiness of their marriage on children's desires to marry and have children were assessed. A stratified random sample of 242 young adults was selected. Results indicated that perceived marital satisfaction in the parental home was a more significant factor in determining the familial aspirations of young adults than was marital dissolution. This was especially the case in assessing at what age respondents desired to get married or start having children. Further, while those from divorced homes did not differ from those from intact homes, those from widowed homes were less likely to aspire to have children.

Marion C. Willetts-Bloom, MA, completed this manuscript as part of a Masters Thesis in the Department of Sociology at the University of Virginia. She is currently affiliated with the National Board of Medical Examiners, 3930 Chestnut Street, Philadelphia, PA 19104.

Steven L. Nock is Associate Professor in the Department of Sociology at the University of Virginia, Charlottesville, VA 22903.

The authors acknowledge the assistance of Paul W. Kingston in proposal formulation, survey construction, and comments on drafts of this paper; Lance C. Bloom in data collection and comments on drafts of this paper, and Marian Borg for comments on a draft of this paper.

© 1992 by The Haworth Press, Inc. All rights reserved.

INTRODUCTION

The well-documented increase in divorce rates over the last thirty years (Toliver, 1986; Beaujot, 1988; Kitagawa, 1981; Kobrin and Waite, 1984) led to much research on the consequences of parental divorce. Much of that research has focused on the economic and social costs of marital disruption (see Weitzman, 1985 and Garfinkel and McLanahan, 1986 for discussions of consequences). One consequence that has received a good deal of attention is the intergenerational transmission of divorce: parents who divorce are more likely to have children who will also divorce than are parents whose marriages remained intact. The effect of parents' divorce on offsprings' chances of divorce has been found consistently, though the strength of the relationship is only weak to moderate (Booth et al., 1984; Greenberg and Nay, 1982; Amato, 1983; Booth and Edwards, 1989; Mueller and Pope, 1977; Kulka and Weingarten, 1979; Pope and Mueller, 1979; Keith and Finlay, 1988; McLanahan and Bumpass, 1988). Related propositions have been that children of divorce are less likely to ever marry (Kobrin and Waite, 1984), that these children will marry at a younger age (Thornton, 1991; Booth et al., 1984; Glenn and Kramer, 1987; McLanahan and Bumpass, 1988; Keith and Finlay, 1988), and that they will begin childbearing at a younger age (McLanahan and Bumpass, 1988; Michael and Tuma, 1985). Some researchers, however, have found no significant differences between children from intact vs. divorced homes with regard to these behaviors (Hogan, 1978; Thornton, 1991). Still others have found that children from widowed homes resemble those from intact homes on these behaviors (Booth et al., 1984; Mitchell et al., 1989). One of the goals of this research is to aid in the clarification of these conflicting findings.

While the results discussed above are of interest, the relationships ignore a significant group: those from unbroken but *unhappy* homes. Although these individuals would be classified as coming from intact homes, it is questionable whether they should be treated in the same way as those from happy, intact families. Several studies have employed measures assessing the degree of conflict in "family of origin" homes. Many of these studies assess effects of parental marital discord on children's future family formation behavior. For example, Scanzoni and Scanzoni (1976) state that many people desiring to be childless came from unhappy, intact homes (also see Booth and Edwards, 1989). Also, according to Thornton (1991), those who came from happy homes are less likely to hurry into marriage to escape an unhappy family setting. Other conclusions in this type of research indicate that children would be better off emotionally if the parents obtained a divorce and ended (or at least significantly reduced) the amount of conflict in the home (Booth et al., 1984; Kurdek and Siesky, 1980; Demo and Acock, 1988). While research on the effects of unhappy home environments is less abundant than that on family structure (i.e., the number and marital status of adults), most authors agree that the level of conflict in the child's home may be more important than structure, and some of these authors state that structure may actually be irrelevant in predicting the child's future family formation behavior (Booth et al., 1984; Demo and Acock, 1988; Booth and Edwards, 1989; Greenberg and Nay, 1982).

The purpose of this research is to investigate the relative effects of childhood family structure and perceptions of parental marital happiness on marital and parenting aspirations. A popular notion among the general population (as well as among many researchers and therapists) has been that divorce has many extremely negative consequences for the children involved, and that parents should "stay together for the sake of the children." Ongoing conflict in the home has not been viewed as negatively as divorce.

While a good deal of disparity exists between aspirations and subsequent behavior, both are important indicators of adjustment to past and current events in one's family of origin. Studying aspirations allows for a more direct test of how childhood events affect current attitudes, without the intervening (and biasing) effects of one's own family formation behavior. Thus, we sought a population of persons of "family formation age." For them, issues of marriage and parenting should be most salient. Second, we sought persons who had not actually started a family, or gotten married. This criterion was imposed to limit any potentially biasing effects of the respondent's current (family) situations discussed above. Third, we desired respondents who were no longer living in their parents' home. In short, our goal was to study the enduring effects of family background on desires and attitudes about family life among individuals no longer living in their families of origin, but not yet in their own families. Non-commuting college students met these requirements. In this research, therefore, college students are not only convenient, but actually a very appropriate group.

HYPOTHESES

Several hypotheses were generated. First, there should be no significant differences among children from intact, widowed, or divorced homes in their aspirations to marry and have children. This is consistent with past research, which shows that most people want children and a spouse (Kinnaird and Gerrard, 1986; Kitagawa, 1981). Because of the conflicting findings in the review, no specific hypotheses were formulated about how childhood family structure would impact on when people want to get married, start childrearing, or the number of children desired, though these are investigated as possible effects of parents' family structure.

Second, there should be a positive relationship between viewing one's parents' marriage as happy and aspiring to marriage and parenting. Furthermore, there should be an inverse relationship between the perceived happiness of one's parents' marriage and desired ages for marriage and start of childrearing. As was stated earlier, Thornton (1991) suggested that early marriage may be in part a result of children wishing to escape the conflictual home of their parents. Here, it was assumed that because the respondents had already left home to go to college, an early marriage as an alternative escape route would be unnecessary. Also, it was hypothesized that there should be a positive relationship between the number of children desired and perceptions of parental marital happiness. Those respondents who viewed their parents' marriage as happy would aspire to more children than would respondents who viewed their parents' marriage as unhappy.

Finally, other background variables were employed as controls. These were: family income, religious preference (collapsed into five categories: Protestant, Catholic, Jewish, other, and none), and frequency of attendance at religious services. Analyses were conducted to compare males and females and whites and non-whites (mainly consisting of blacks and Asian/Asian-Americans). Results were considered statistically significant at the $p \leq .10$ level. We used this liberal level of significance because our sample was small and our measures (for which there are no existing validated indicators) are crude.

DATA AND METHODS

Procedure

College students were chosen as the sample because it was assumed that family issues are more salient for this age group than for nearly any other. Furthermore, because this is a very homogeneous population in important respects, other background effects could be more easily controlled.

A random sample stratified by year in school (four years) of 500 undergraduate students living on campus at a moderate-sized public university in Virginia was drawn. Printed surveys were distributed through the university postal system to 495 undergraduates [five were dropped from the initial list due to withdrawal from the university (3) and non-existent addresses (2)]. Each survey was assigned a number which corresponded to a Master List of names. After four weeks, a follow-up survey was sent to those who had yet to respond. A total response rate of 49% was obtained (242 cases).

Subjects

Eighty-one percent of the respondents in the sample were from intact homes, with 12.8% from homes broken by divorce and 4.5% from homes broken by death. Almost 44% viewed their parents' marriage as very happy, while nearly 40% and 17% viewed their parents' marriage as pretty happy or not happy at all (respectively). Respondent's age at time of parental marital disruption, with whom the respondent was living at age 16, and how frequently the respondent saw the non-custodial parent were all found to be insignificant factors in the analyses, and thus will not be elaborated on here.

Among the respondents, there were 111 males (46% of total) and 131 females (54%). White students comprised 74% of the sample, with blacks forming 14.5% and the remaining 11.5% falling into the initial "other" category (these latter two were combined in subsequent analyses). The modal category of religious preference was Protestant (46.9%), followed by those claiming no religious preference (19.9%), Catholics (19.1%), other religious preferences (10.8%), and Jews (3.3%). For attendance at religious services, the modal category was "several times a year" (22.8%), with the remainder normally distributed on a continuum ranging from "never" to "several times a week." As was expected for residential college students, total family income was often high: less than 25% of the sample stated that their total family income was under $35,000 per year, and approximately 17% of the sample stated that their total family income was $100,000 or more per year (see Appendix 1 for coding of all variables).

Dependent Variables

The dependent variables employed in these analyses included the following: (1) First, respondents were asked to indicate whether or not they desired to marry in their futures (96.2% expressed such a desire). (2) Respondents who desired to marry were then asked to indicate at what age they would prefer to marry ($\bar{x} = 26.013$, s = 2.531). (3) Then, respondents also indicated whether or not they desired to have children (91.9% expressed such a desire). (4) Those who desired to have children then noted at what age they would prefer to begin childbearing ($\bar{x} = 28.404$, s = 2.692). (5) Finally, respondents who desired children then specified how many children they planned to have ($\bar{x} = 2.661$, s = 1.143).

Independent Variables

The independent variables used in these analyses included the following: (1) Respondents were asked to state their parents' marital status when they were sixteen years old. All respondents but one indicated that their parents had either an intact marriage (81%), or one broken by divorce or death (17.3%). The one respondent who indicated that the parents never married was excluded. (2) Respondents were asked who they were living with at age sixteen. Eighty-one percent of the sample indicated that they were living with both their own parents at age 16. Another 10.7% stated that they were living with only their mother. One respondent indicated that he was living with only his father. Approximately 4% claimed that they were living with both their mothers and their stepfathers at age 16, while 2.5% stated that they were living with their fathers and their stepmothers at this age. Finally, 1.2% of the sample indicated that they were living under some other type of arrangement (typically with other relatives). No significant results were obtained by using this variable, and will thus not be discussed further. (3) Those not living with both parents were asked to indicate how frequently they saw (visited, etc.) the non-custodial parent at age sixteen. The modal response was "less than once a year" (41%). The next most popular choice was "several times a month" (17.4%). Approximately 11% selected the response of "once a week." The rest were relatively evenly distributed among the other possible choices, ranging from "more than once a week" to "once every six months to one year." No significant findings were obtained in analyses employing this variable either. (4) Respondents also expressed how long they had lived with both their own parents by age sixteen. This variable was collapsed into three categories (0 to 5 years, 6 to 10 years, and 11 to 16 years). Over 84% of the sample stated that they lived with both parents for 11 to 16 years. Furthermore, 7.5% selected the 6 to 10 years category, and 8.3% selected the 0 to 5 years category. Again, no significant findings were obtained here. (5) Finally, a variable was employed to measure respondent's perceptions of the marital happiness of the parental home. Here, we are not presuming to measure the parents' *actual* marital happiness, but rather the respondents' *perceptions* of the marriage. Also, we desired a measure which would express the overall perceptions of the marriage, rather than a specific point of time in the marriage. For example, asking the respondent to assess the parents' marital happiness at say, age 16, would be inappropriate in several instances: one, the marriage may have been dissolved by that time, so there would be no marriage to assess; or two, an incident may have occurred at that time reference which was generally atypical of the marriage, but impacted on it for a time (e.g., long-term unemployment). So, respondents were asked to respond to the following: "Taking all things together, how would you describe your parents' marriage?" The possible response choices were very happy, pretty happy, and not happy at all. This measure is comparable to that employed by Amato and Booth (1991). Crosstabular analyses were conducted to determine how those from differing family structures responded to this question. A significant, moderate relationship was found (X^2 = 80.308, p = .0000; Cramer's V = .416, lambda = .16). Fifty percent of those from intact homes viewed their parents' marriage as very happy (30% from widowed homes and 3.6% from divorced homes reported as such), while 41.8% from intact homes viewed their parents' marriage as pretty happy (50% from widowed homes; 21.4% from divorced homes) and 8.2% from intact homes viewed their parents' marriage as not at all happy (20% from widowed homes and 75% from divorced homes selected this category). Thus, parents' marital status is correlated with perceptions about the happiness of their marriage (as would be expected). However, there is sufficient variation to allow us to investigate the independent effects of these two factors.

RESULTS

Marital Aspirations

Plans to marry. Since this variable is a dichotomy, logistic regression analysis was conducted with plans to marry as the dependent variable (results for the analysis of intentions to marry are shown in the left-hand panel of Table 1). The regression coefficient is the change in the log-odds of marital plans for a one-unit change in the variable. The second column (Exp (b)) expresses these effects as changes in "odds." A value of 1.0 means the variable does not affect the odds, a value of greater than 1.0 means the variable increases the odds, and a value of less than 1.0 means the odds are reduced. There was very little variance in the dependent variable since the vast majority of the sample plans to marry (96.2%). Still, the model was significant (p = .0505). Parents' marital status did not significantly affect respondents' aspirations to marry, as was expected. Furthermore, perceptions of parents' marital happiness was also insignificant in determining who aspired to marry. Again, because such a large majority planned to marry, these variables were not expected to be significant.

Several control variables did emerge as important. A student's race was a significant predictor of plans to marry (p = .0128). Non-whites were less likely to aspire to marriage than were whites, controlling for all other variables in the model (B = –2.2172).

The regression coefficient for RACE (–2.2172) (or any other variable) can be re-expressed in terms of its effects on the *odds* of intending to marry. Whereas the regression (logistic) coefficient of –2.2172 can be interpreted as the change in the *log* odds due to race, it is easier to think in terms of *odds*. This can be done by raising e (the base of the natural logarithms) to B = –2.2172. The result is the amount the odds of intending to marry differ due to race. In this case, $e^{-2.2172}$ corresponds to a difference in the odds of intending to marry of a factor of .10 due to race.

To understand the meaning of this figure, consider the odds of intending to marry for two persons alike on all variables *except* race: specifically, two individuals from parents with intact marriages (PARDIVOR = 0, PARDIED = 0) who viewed their parents' marriage as happy (MARPAR = 2), who are of "other" or no religious affiliations (CATHOLIC = 0, JEWISH = 0, OTHER/ NONE = 1), who attend religious services once a month (ATTEND = 12), who are male (SEX = 1) with parents' income in the $25,000–$30,000 range (INCOME = 10). Race is coded 1 for whites and 2 for nonwhites.

First, we can calculate the probability that a white student like this intends to marry by applying the coefficients from Table 1 to the values of the appropriate variables. Thus, the estimated probability (that a student intends to marry) is equal to $1/1 + e^{-z}$, where z = 2.4866 (CONSTANT) + .5956*2 (.5956 is the regression coefficient for MARPAR, 2 is the value of MARPAR) – 1.7752*1 (OTHER/NONE = 1) + .5090*12 (ATTEND) + –2.2172*1 (RACE) + .3277*1 (SEX) + .0961*10 (INCOME) = 7.0821. So, the estimated probability that a white student intends to marry is $1/1 + e^{-7.0821}$ = .9992. Using the same procedure for a black student (the only

TABLE 1

Regression Analysis of Intention to Marry and Desired
Age at Marriage on Family Background Variables

Independent Variables:	INTEND TO MARRY (0=NO, 1=YES)+		AGE AT MARRIAGE++	
	Regression Coefficient	Exp(b)	b	beta
PARDIVOR (parents divorced)	-1.0189	.3610	-.18291	-.02222
PARDIED (parent died)	-1.4911	.2251	.03985	.00278
PARBOTH (intact marriage)	deleted		deleted	
MARPAR (parents' marital happiness 1=very,3=not happy)	.5956	1.8141	.59181**	.16192
RELIGION:				
CATHOLIC	-.4887	.6134	.87850*	.13770
JEWISH	-2.2869	.1016	.62118	.04341
OTHER/NONE	-1.7752**	.1694	.22290	.03734
PROTESTANT	deleted		deleted	
ATTEND (church attendance times/year)	.5090**	1.6636	-.17585**	-.1566
RACE (1=W, 2=NW)	-2.2172***	.1089	1.3314****	.2201
SEX (respondent's sex 1=M,2=F)	.3277	1.3878	-.49364	-.09483
INCOME (total family income)	.0961	1.1009	.02325	.02869
Constant	2.4866		24.37292	

(Table notes appear on following page)

TABLE 1 (continued)

```
+LOGISTIC REGRESSION
++OLS REGRESSION
*  p < .10    ***  p < .01
**p < .05    **** p < .0001

INTEND TO MARRY EQUATION STATISTICS:
                        Chi-Square     Df     Significance
-2 Log Likelihood         56.634      206        1.0000
Model Chi-Square          18.276       10         .0505
Improvement               18.276       10         .0505
Goodness of Fit          126.043      206        1.0000

AGE AT MARRIAGE EQUATION STATISTICS:

R²  =    .11118
F   =   2.43931        Sig  =   .0092
N   =    205
```

difference being that the value for RACE is 2.0) yields z = 4.8649 for an estimated probability of .9924. Clearly, students of both races have extremely high probabilities of intending to marry. The *odds* of intending to marry for whites are calculated as [.9992/(1 −.9992)] = 1249; and for blacks [.9924/(1 −.9924)] = 131. So by changing the value of RACE from 1 to 2 (white to black) the *odds* of intending to marry changed from 1249 to 131. That is, they decreased by a factor of .105 (i.e., 131/1249); the figure shown in the column labelled Exp (B) in Table 1 (shown there as .1089 rather than .105; a difference due to rounding).

Attendance at religious services was also found to significantly increase the reported desire to marry (p = .0258). The odds of intending to marry for those who reported the highest rate of attendance (several times per week) were greater by a factor of .66 than were those for students who attended once per week. This variable was also moderate in strength (Bivariate R = .1990). Some of the religious preference variables were also significant, with Protestants serving as the reference group. Here, those claiming no religious preference and other religious preferences were combined into one category, and dummy variables were constructed. Only those claiming no or other religious preferences differed significantly from Protestants (p = .0476). Those claiming no or other religious preferences were less likely to express a desire to marry. No other variables in the model were significant.

Age at marriage. Respondents were asked to indicate at what age they would prefer to marry (results for this variable are shown in Columns 3 and 4 in Table 1). The modal choice was 25, and the range was ages twenty to thirty-seven. Since this variable is continuous, OLS multiple regression was used. The model was significant (p = .0092, r^2 = .11). We see that perceptions of parental marital happiness influence the aspired-to age at marriage (b = .592). Those who viewed their parents' marriage as unhappy aspired to later ages at marriage. The size of this coefficient suggests that two respondents identical on other variables but differing by two points on the perceived parental marital happiness variable would differ by (2*.59) = 1.18 years in the ages they intend to marry. As was found for intentions to marry, parental marital status had no significant effects on age at which respondents plan to marry.

Race was also found to influence the age at which students intend to marry. Non-whites reported an intended age at marriage that was 1.33 years *later* than whites (p < .001). Furthermore, frequent attendance at religious services was found to be associated with younger ages at which marriage was expected (b = −.176). Finally, only Catholics differed from Protestants on this measure: Catholics reported a somewhat older age for marriage (almost one year; b = .878).

While perceptions of parents' marital happiness were found to be related to one measure of familial aspirations (i.e., intended age at first marriage, but not intentions to marry), parental family structure was related to neither. Perceptions about parents' marriages played a significant role in the desired age at marriage, but family structure did not. Furthermore, other variables such as race, religious preference, and attendance (in both plans to marry and desired ages) contributed to the understanding of marital aspirations.

Parenting Aspirations

Intentions to become a parent. As was expected, the majority of the sample plans to have children (91.9%) and logistic regression was employed, with plans to have children coded as a dichotomous variable (see left panel of Table 2). The model was significant (p = .0060). On this measure, those from widowed homes differed significantly from those from intact homes (p = .0829). Those from widowed homes were much less likely to aspire to having children (b = –1.71; Exp (b) = .18). However, students from divorced homes did not differ significantly from those from intact homes in this model. Most importantly, perceptions of parents' marital happiness had no significant effects on parental plans.

The only other significant variable in this model was frequency of attendance at religious services (p = .0046). Those who attend services more frequently expressed a greater desire to have children (b = .4434; Exp (b) = 1.56).

Desired age at parenthood. Respondents were asked to indicate the age at which they plan to begin childbearing. The modal choice was age 28, and the range was 22 to 40. Multiple regression analysis (OLS) was used, and the model was significant (p = .0693, r^2 = .09). Again, parents' marital status had no significant effects (see Table Two). Perceptions of parents' marital happiness, however, did emerge as significant: those who perceived their parents' marriage as unhappy reported later ages for childbearing. Two respondents identical on other variables but differing by two points on their perceptions of their parents' marital happiness would differ by an estimated (2*.81) = 1.62 years in the ages they intend to begin having children.

Sex was also found to be significant: females reported younger desired ages to start childbearing than did males, by about .8 years (as was expected).

Desired number of children. Respondents were also asked to indicate how many children they hoped to have (results not shown). The modal choice was two children, chosen by 48.9% of the sample. The range was one child to nine children (for those who wanted children at all). The model was significant (p < .0010; r^2 = .14). Interestingly, both the family structure variables and the perception variable were both insignificant (thus, the equation is summarized here, rather than presented in Table 2). Family income was significant, suggesting that those from higher income families desired fewer children. Attendance at religious services was also significant showing that more frequent attendance was associated with a desire

TABLE 2

Regression Analysis of Intention to Have Children and Desired Age at Start of Childbearing on Family Background Variables

Independent Variables:	INTEND TO HAVE CHILDREN+ (0=NO, 1=YES) Regression Coefficient	Exp(b)	AGE AT CHILD-BEARING++ b	beta
PARDIVOR (parents divorced)	1.7286	5.6330	-.00330	-.0004
PARDIED (parent died)	-1.7064*	.1815	-.24100	-.01413
PARBOTH (intact marriage)	deleted		deleted	
MARPAR (parents' marital happiness)	-.6140	.5412	.80981***	.21526
RELIGION:				
CATHOLIC	1.0354	2.8161	-.27370	-.04166
JEWISH	-1.0002	.3678	-.54858	-.03514
OTHER/NONE	.4018	1.4945	-.35673	-.05606
PROTESTANT	deleted		deleted	
ATTEND (attendance at services)	.4434***	1.5580	-.14896	-.12746
RACE (1=W,2=NW)	-.2045	.8150	.48598	.07853
SEX (1=M,2=F)	.5314	1.7012	-.75847**	-.13854
INCOME (total family income)	.0736	1.0763	.04308	.05272
Constant	.2423		27.88924	

(Table notes appear on following page)

TABLE 2 (continued)

```
+LOGISTIC REGRESSION
++OLS REGRESSION
*   p < .10                    *** p <.01
**  p < .05                    **** p < .001
```

INTEND TO HAVE CHILDREN EQUATION STATISTICS:

	Chi-Square	Df	Significance
-2 Log Likelihood	99.570	207	1.0000
Model Chi-Square	24.690	10	.0060
Improvement	24.690	10	.0060
Goodness of Fit	190.272	207	.7917

AGE AT CHILDBEARING EQUATION STATISTICS:

```
R²  =    .08899
F   =  1.76811      Sig  =  .0693
N   =  191
```

for a larger number of children (b = .0795). With Protestants as the reference group, Catholics expressed a desire for about one more child than did Protestants (b = .79). Also, students claiming other or no religious affiliation desired slightly more children than did Protestants (b = .45).

To summarize the parenting variables, it appears that neither childhood family structure nor perceptions of parents' marital happiness are important factors in determining whether or not students desire to become parents. Those from widowed homes were somewhat less likely than those from intact homes to aspire to having children. But those from divorced homes did not differ significantly from those from intact homes on this measure. And, while the overwhelming majority of students reported a desire to become parents eventually, those who perceived their parents' marriage as less happy desired a later age at the start of childbearing (as was expected). Finally, neither family structure nor perceptions of parents' marital happiness significantly affected the desired number of children.

DISCUSSION

This research has identified several significant effects of both childhood family structure and perceptions of parents' marriage on young peoples' familial aspirations. The hypothesis that none of the parental marital status groups would differ in their desire to marry was supported. Also, the hypothesis that perceptions of parental marital happiness would influence the desired age at marriage was supported. Those who viewed their parents' marriage as unhappy appeared more cautious in their own marital aspirations, reporting a later desired age at marriage. There were no differences among those from intact, widowed, or divorced families on this measure. It appears in this case that those from divorced homes in particular overcame the negative effects of the disruption.

Also, the hypothesis that perceptions of parental marital happiness would be a significant predictor in determining desired ages at start of parenting was supported, again in the expected direction.

However, several hypotheses did not receive support. It was expected that there would be no differences among any of the parental marital status groups in reported desires to have children. However, those from widowed homes were less likely to desire children than were those from intact homes. One possible explanation for this finding may be that these children feel more obligated to the widowed parent, making the assumption of parental duties appear more onerous. Another possibility is a fear of widowhood in their own marriages and the negative effects such an experience might have on the children.

Furthermore, we expected that viewing one's parents' marriage as happy would increase desires for marriage and parenthood. We found, however, that such perceptions played no role in such desires.

For several key issues in this research, neither family structure nor perceptions of parental marital happiness was a significant influence. We are left to wonder whether this might be because the respondents in our study have overcome the possible negative consequences of divorce discussed in previous literature. Since these children were able to attend college, we may assume that some of the economic effects of divorce typically found in the general population may not be so salient. This may also be the case for those from widowed homes. Further, our respondents were able to leave conflictual homes by going to college. Thus, they may feel less urgency to escape an unhappy home life by starting families of their own, while such a strategy may be more attractive to those with fewer options.

To summarize, the perceptions of parental marital happiness in the home appeared to be a more significant factor in young peoples' familial aspirations than was the structure of their childhood home. This conclusion was mainly true in determining *when* the respondents desired to get married and have children. However, future research should examine these relationships with a more heterogeneous population. Also, other background variables should be employed, and more measures of each variable should be constructed. For example, the respondent's perceptions of how happy his/her childhood was would most likely prove fruitful in this type of research. Number of siblings and placement in the birth order may also provide interesting results. Furthermore, types of support from other family members, friends, neighbors, etc. in cases of divorce and widowhood would shed much light on the processes involved in adjustment to the new situations, particularly since (as was stated earlier) respondent's age at time of disruption and degree of contact with the non-custodial parent were insignificant predictors of familial aspirations in this research. If family members or other role models served as "substitutes" for the absent parent, socialization lessons that conform more or less to society's norms may have continued with little interruption. In addition, the types of conflict in the parental home may be significant. Whatever direction other studies take, the effects of family of origin structure and perceptions of parents' marital happiness on aspirations justify future exploration.

REFERENCES

Amato, Paul R. 1988. "Parental Divorce and Attitudes Toward Marriage and Family Life." Journal of Marriage and the Family 50: 453-461.

Amato, Paul R. and Alan Booth. "Consequences of Parental Divorce and Marital Unhappiness for Adult Well-Being." Social Forces 69: 895-914.

Booth, Alan, David B. Brinkerhoff, and Lynn K. White. 1984. "The Impact of Parental Divorce on Courtship." Journal of Marriage and the Family 46: 85-94.

Booth, Alan and John N. Edwards. 1989. "Transmission of Marital and Family Quality Over the Generations." Journal of Divorce 13: 41-58.

Demo, David H. and Alan C. Acock. 1988. "The Impact of Divorce on Children." Journal of Marriage and the Family 50: 619-648.

Garfinkel, Irwin and Sara S. McLanahan. 1986. Single Mothers and Their Children: A New American Dilemma. Washington, D. C.: The Urban Institute.

Glenn, Norval D. and Kathryn B. Kramer. 1987. "The Marriages and Divorces of the Children of Divorce." Journal of Marriage and the Family 49: 811-825.

Greenberg, Ellen F. and W. Robert Nay. 1982. "The Intergenerational Transmission of Marital Instability Reconsidered." Journal of Marriage and the Family 44: 335-347.

Hogan, Dennis P. 1978. "The Effects of Demographic Factors, Family Background, and Early Job Achievement on Age at Marriage." Demography 15: 161-175.

Keith, Verna M. and Barbara Finlay. 1988. "The Impact of Parental Divorce on Children's Educational Attainment, Marital Timing, and Likelihood of Divorce." Journal of Marriage and the Family 50: 797-809.

Kinnaird, Keri L. and Meg Gerrard. 1986. "Premarital Sexual Behavior and Attitudes Toward Marriage and Divorce Among Young Women as a Function of Their Mothers' Marital Status." Journal of Marriage and the Family 48: 757-765.

Kitagawa, Evelyn M. 1981. "New Life-Styles: Marriage Patterns, Living Arrangements, and Fertility Outside of Marriage." The Annals of the American Academy of Political and Social Science 453: 1-27.

Kobrin, Frances E. and Linda J. Waite. 1984. "Effects of Childhood Family Structure on the Transition to Marriage." Journal of Marriage and the Family 46: 907-916.

Kulka, Richard A. and Helen Weingarten. 1979. "The Long-Term Effects of Parental Divorce in Childhood on Adult Adjustment." Journal of Social Issues 35: 50-78.

Kurdek, Lawrence A. and Albert E. Siesky, Jr. 1980. "Children's Perceptions of Their Parents' Divorce." Journal of Divorce 3: 339-378.

McLanahan, Sara and Larry Bumpass. 1988. "Intergenerational Consequences of Family Disruption." American Journal of Sociology 94: 130-152.

Michael, Robert T. and Nancy Brandon Tuma. 1985. "Entry Into Marriage and Parenthood by Young Men and Women: The Influence of Family Background." Demography 22: 515-544.

Mitchell, Barbara A., Andrew V. Wister, and Thomas K. Burch. 1989. "The Family Environment and Leaving the Parental Home." Journal of Marriage and the Family 51: 605-613.

Mueller, Charles W. and Hallowell Pope. 1977. "Marital Instability: A Study of Its Transmission Between Generations." Journal of Marriage and the Family 39: 83-93.

National Opinion Research Center. 1988. General Social Surveys, 1972-1988: Cumulative Codebook. Chicago, IL: National Opinion Research Center.

Pope, Hallowell and Charles W. Mueller. 1976. "The Intergenerational Transmission of Marital Instability: Comparisons by Race and Sex." Journal of Social Issues 32: 49-66.

Scanzoni, Letha and John Scanzoni. 1976. Men, Women, and Change: A Sociology of Marriage and the Family. USA: McGraw-Hill Book Company, Inc.

Thornton, Arland. 1991. "Influence of the Marital History of Parents on the Marital and Cohabitational Experiences of Children." American Journal of Sociology 96: 868-894.

Weitzman, Lenore J. 1985. The Divorce Revolution: The Unexpected Social and Economic Consequences for Women and Children in America. New York: The Free Press.

APPENDIX I

Coding of Variables Used in Analyses

```
PLNMAR    (plans to marry)
          0 = NO
          1 = YES

AGEMAR    (preferred age at marriage)
          continuous variable

PLNKID    (plans to have children)
          0 = NO
          1 = YES

AGEKID    (preferred age at start of childbearing)
          continuous variable

NUMKID    (preferred number of children)
          continuous variable

PARDIVOR  (parents divorced)
          0 = NO
          1 = YES

PARDIED   (parent died)
          0 = NO
          1 = YES

PARBOTH   (intact marriage of parents)
          0 = NO
          1 = YES

FAMBACK   (years living with both parents to age 16)
          1 = 0 TO 5 YEARS
          2 = 6 TO 10 YEARS
          3 = 11 TO 16 YEARS
```

APPENDIX (continued)

WHOLIV   (who R lived with, if not both one's own
          parents)
          1 = FATHER AND STEPMOTHER
          2 = MOTHER AND STEPFATHER
          3 = FATHER ONLY
          4 = MOTHER ONLY
          5 = SOME OTHER MALE RELATIVE
          6 = SOME OTHER FEMALE RELATIVE
          7 = OTHER ARRANGEMENT WITH RELATIVES (E.G.,
              GRANDPARENTS, AUNT AND UNCLE, ETC.)
          8 = OTHER

FREQPAR   (how frequently R saw non-custodial parent)
          1 = MORE THAN ONCE A WEEK
          2 = ONCE A WEEK
          3 = SEVERAL TIMES A MONTH
          4 = ONCE A MONTH
          5 = ONCE EVERY TWO OR THREE MONTHS
          6 = ONCE EVERY FOUR TO SIX MONTHS
          7 = ONCE EVERY SIX MONTHS TO ONE YEAR
          8 = LESS THAN ONCE A YEAR

MARPAR   (parents' marital happiness)
          1 = VERY HAPPY
          2 = PRETTY HAPPY
          3 = NOT HAPPY AT ALL

RELIGION (R's religious affiliation)
          CATHOLIC
            0 = NO
            1 = YES
          PROTESTANT
            0 = NO
            1 = YES
          JEWISH
            0 = NO
            1 = YES
          OTHER/NONE
            0 = NO
            1 = YES

ATTEND   (R's frequency of attendance at religious
          services)
          0   = NEVER
          1   = LESS THAN ONCE A YEAR
          2   = ABOUT ONCE OR TWICE A YEAR
          6   = SEVERAL TIMES A YEAR
          12 = ABOUT ONCE A MONTH
          30 = TWO TO THREE TIMES A MONTH
          44 = NEARLY EVERY WEEK
          52 = EVERY WEEK
          104 = SEVERAL TIMES A WEEK

```
RACE        (R's race)
            1 = WHITE
            2 = NON-WHITE

SEX         (R's sex)
            1 = MALE
            2 = FEMALE

INCOME      (total annual family income)
            1  = UNDER $1,000
            2  = $1,000 TO $4,999
            3  = $5,000 TO $7,499
            4  = $7,500 TO $9,999
            5  = $10,000 TO $12,499
            6  = $12,500 TO $14,999
            7  = $15,000 TO $17,499
            8  = $17,500 TO $19,999
            9  = $20,000 TO $24,999
            10 = $25,000 TO $29,999
            11 = $30,000 TO $34,999
            12 = $35,000 TO $39,999
            13 = $40,000 TO $49,999
            14 = $50,000 TO $59,999
            15 = $60,000 TO $74,999
            16 = $75,000 TO $99,999
            17 = $100,000 AND OVER
```

Intimate Relationships:
College Students from Divorced
and Intact Families

Lisa Gabardi
Lee A. Rosén

SUMMARY. The study examined differences between college students from divorced and intact families on several measures of intimate relationships. Analyses indicated that students from divorced families had more sexual partners and desired more sexual involvement when going steady than students from intact families. Regression analyses indicated that, for students from both divorced and intact families, parental marital conflict was a significant predictor of total number of sexual partners and negative attitudes toward marriage. In addition, parents' marital status was a significant predictor of sexual involvement while going steady and a significant predictor of self perceptions of sociability and morality. For students from divorced families, conflict after the divorce was a significant predictor of sexual involvement while going steady and negative attitudes toward marriage. Number of years since the divorce occurred was also a significant predictor of sexual involvement desired after several dates, relationship beliefs, and attitudes toward marriage for students from divorced families. Implications of these results are discussed in terms of college students' development of intimate relationships.

Investigators have recently begun to study the effects of parental divorce on adult "children" of divorce. Although research has indicated that age and developmental stage are critical factors affecting young children's response to divorce (Hetherington, 1981; Krudek,

Lisa Gabardi, PhD, is currently a licensed psychologist at the Delaunay Mental Health Center in Portland, OR. Lee Rosén, PhD, is Associate Professor in the Department of Psychology, Colorado State University, Fort Collins, CO 80523.

© 1992 by The Haworth Press, Inc. All rights reserved.

1981; Wallerstein & Kelly, 1980) few investigations have focused on the impact of parental divorce on measures relevant to the developmental stage of adult children. Many researchers have continued to focus on measures of adjustment used in studies with younger children-psychological adjustment, academic success, sexrole development, self-concept, family relations, and loss (Farber, Primavera, & Felner, 1983; Fine, Moreland, & Schwebel, 1983; Grossman, Shea, & Adams, 1980; Kulka, Weingarten, 1979). The effects parental divorce may have on young adult issues such as dating, sexuality, ability to be intimate, and beliefs about relationships and marriage have not been adequately examined (Booth, Brinkerhoff, & White, 1984; Hepworth, Ryder, & Dreyer, 1984; Hillard, 1984; Kalter, Riember, Buckman, & Woo Chen, 1985; Kelly, 1981). Some researchers have suggested that young adults from divorced families differ from those of intact families in their beliefs and behaviors involving intimate relationships (Cooney, Smyer, Hagestad, Klock, 1986; Parish, 1981; Vess, Schwebel, & Moreland, 1983). We conducted this study to expand our understanding of how intimacy development is impacted by parental divorce.

METHOD

Subjects

Subjects were 300 college students enrolled in introductory psychology courses at Colorado State University. To decrease the demographic variance of the subject pool, only students who were between 18 and 25 years of age, single, heterosexual, had parents that were still married or had been divorced only once, and had not been sexually abused were included in the study.[1] Information on the demographic characteristics of the subject pool is presented in Table 1.

Procedure

Students were pre-screened to meet the demographic criteria for this study using the demographic data sheet. Subjects from divorced

Table 1

Demographic Characteristics of the Subject Pool

Characteristic	N	Percent (%)
Gender		
Female	193	64.3
Male	107	35.7
Race/Ethnicity		
Asian American	22	3.7
Black	12	4.0
Caucasian	255	85.0
Hispanic	16	5.3
Native American	4	1.3
Other (Unspecified)	2	0.7
Religion		
Catholic	97	32.3
Christian	76	25.3
Jewish	12	4.0
Protestant	57	19.0
Agnostic	23	7.7
Other (Unspecified)	31	11.6
Class Standing		
Freshman	171	57.0
Sophomore	44	14.7
Junior	56	18.7
Senior	28	9.3
Other	1	0.3
Parental Marital Status		
Married	185	61.7
Divorced	115	38.3

and intact families were randomly selected from the pre-screening information. Subjects were then asked to complete a series of paper and pencil questionnaires regarding demographic information, dating status, sexual behaviors, relationship beliefs, intimacy, attitudes toward marriage, and self-esteem. Surveys were group administered and all subjects were informed that the survey information was completely confidential. Questionnaires in the survey packets were randomly ordered and identified by subject number to maintain anonymity.

Measures

Demographic data sheet. Subjects completed a series of questions regarding age, gender, marital status, religion, racial/ethnic background, class, grade point average and academic major, and family information such as parental education. Subjects were also asked several questions regarding their biological parents' marital history.

Parental conflict scale. Subjects were asked to rate the level of conflict between their parents on a Likert scale from 1 to 7 (1 = no conflict, 7 = extremely high conflict). If students' parents were divorced, students were also asked to rate the conflict between their parents for the year prior to the divorce and for the year following the divorce on a similar Likert scale. While this scale is based upon students' recollections of their parents' relationships, we felt it was important to assess how students perceived their parents' relationship when they were growing up. Some researchers suggest that students' perceptions of their parents' relationship are more pertinent to their adjustment than their parents' actual level of conflict (Greenberg & Nay, 1982).

Sexual Behavior Measures

Sexuality inventory. Subjects were asked questions regarding their dating status, frequency of their current and past sexual behavior, and sexual orientation. Subjects were asked to report the age at which they first engaged in sexual intercourse and the frequency in which they engage in a series of sexual behaviors. Behaviors included: light and heavy petting, oral sex, and sexual intercourse. If the subject had engaged in sexual intercourse, s/he was asked to report the total number of partners. This inventory is based on a sampling of items from the Heterosexual Behavior Assessment Scale (Bentler, 1968) and the Premarital Sexual Permissiveness Scale (Reiss, 1967).

Depth of Sexual Involvement Scale. The Depth of Sexual Involvement Scales (SIS) is a twelve-item, Guttman-type selfreport measure of behaviors that may be experienced in heterosexual relationships (McCabe & Collins, 1984). Subjects were asked to indicate which of the twelve behaviors they would like to experience in a heterosexual dating relationship and which of the twelve behaviors they actually had experienced in a dating relationship. Responses were made across three stages of dating: first date, several dates, and going steady. Scores were determined by calculating the total number of affirmative responses, the maximum being twelve. Test-retest stability for a norm group of college students, ages 17-19, was .73-.96 (McCabe & Collins, 1984). The coefficient alpha test of internal consistency is high (= .87) (McCabe & Collins, 1984). The scale has strong, though preliminary, evidence of construct and criterion validity (McCabe & Collins, 1984).

Belief and Attitude Measures

Attitudes Toward Marriage. Subjects completed an 8-item Attitudes Toward Marriage Scale designed to measure their current beliefs about marriage (Gabardi & Rosén, 1991). The 8 items are of the Likert type allowing one of four responses from "strongly agree" to "strongly disagree." Items belong to one of the two subscales measuring idealized beliefs or personal doubts about marriage. Items characterizing idealized beliefs included the following: "If I marry, I intend to stay married to my spouse for the rest of my life," and "loving each other is enough to keep a marriage together." Items characterizing personal doubts included: "If I get married, I have little confidence that my marriage will be a success," and "I feel very cautious about entering into a marriage." Items from each scale were scored separately to yield two scale scores. High scores indicated either highly idealized or very apprehensive attitudes about marriage. In addition, a total score of all items was calculated such that a high total score indicated negative attitudes toward marriage. A Chronbach alpha test of internal consistency was performed for each subscale and for the entire scale. The standardized item alpha for the Doubt subscale was 0.69, and for the Ideal subscale alpha equaled 0.59. The standardized item alpha for the entire scale was 0.68, indicating moderately high reliability for the scale.

Relationship Belief Inventory. The Relationship Belief Inventory (RBI) is a forty-item scale designed to assess some of the beliefs about intimate relationships that contribute to distress (Eidelson & Epstein, 1982). The forty items are of the Likert type, allowing for one of five responses from "I strongly believe that the statement is true" to "I strongly believe the statement is false." Total scores were computed for each of five subscales: disagreement is destructive, mindreading is expected, partners cannot change, sexual perfection is expected, and the sexes are different. Items included the following: "I do not expect my partner to sense all of my moods. Men and women probably will never understand the opposite sex very well. A partner that hurts you badly once probably will hurt you again. If you don't like the way a relationship is going, you can make it better." High scale scores indicate many relationship beliefs that contribute to distress. The Chronbach alpha internal consistency coefficients for the five RBI scales range from .72 to .81. Scale scores were significantly and positively correlated to a measure of irrational beliefs about one's self, indicating good concurrent validity (Eidelson & Epstein, 1982). Construct validity has been indicated through significant differences in scale scores for clinic and non-clinic samples of partners in intimate relationships and negative scale score correlations to the Locke-Wallace Marital Adjustment Scale (Eidelson & Epstein, 1982).

Adult Self-Perception Profile. The Adult Self-Perception Profile (HSE) is a fifty-item scale measuring global and domain-specific self-worth (Messer & Harter, 1986). Each item is based on a forced-choice, four-point scale format. Two statements are given per item; one statement representing negative self-worth, the other positive. Subjects were asked to select which statement was most like them and then indicate how true the statement was for them ("really true for me" or "sort of true for me"). In addition to a global self-worth scale, items are divided into eleven specific domains. Each subscale contains four items and the global self-worth scale contains six items. Four subscales were used in this study: Sociability, Morality, Intimate Relationships and Global Self-Worth. Each item was scored from 1 to 4, where 1 indicated low perceived competence/ adequacy and 4 indicated high perceived-competence/adequacy. Internal consistency (Chronbach alpha) ranged from .63 to .91 across the four scales chosen for this study with a norm group of working adult men and women (Messer & Harter, 1986). High factor loadings have also been obtained for each of the subscales chosen for this study (Messer & Harter, 1986).

Rosenberg Self-Esteem Scale. The Rosenberg Self-Esteem scale (RSE) is a ten-item Guttman scale designed to measure global positive or negative attitudes toward one's self (Rosenberg, 1965). The ten items are of the Likert type allowing one of four responses: "strongly agree," "agree," "disagree," "strongly disagree." Items include the following type: "I feel that I have a number of good qualities. All in all, I am inclined to feel that I am a failure. I am able to do things as well as most other people. I feel I do not have much to be proud of." Positively and negatively worded items are in alternate order to reduce response set. A high total score indicates low self-esteem. High self-esteem signifies that the individual respects himself and is worthy. Low self-esteem reflects a lack of self-respect and sense of inadequacy (Johnson, 1976). The scale was normed against 5,024 high school juniors and seniors. Internal reliability is indicated by 92 percent reproducibility and 72 percent scalability. Test-retest reliability with college students was .85. The scale has also been tested for evidence of construct validity (Johnson, 1976; Rosenberg, 1965). The scale is highly correlated with measures of depressive affect and psychophysiological indicators of anxiety (Johnson 1976). In addition, young adults that scored high on the scale (indicating low self-esteem) were described by nurses to be gloomy and frequently disappointed (Johnson, 1976).

Miller Social Intimacy Scale. The Miller Social Intimacy Scale (MSIS) is a 17-item scale designed to measure the maximum level of intimacy experienced in the context of either a friendship or heterosexual dating relationship (Miller & Lefcourt, 1982). Items are scored on a ten-point scale. Six of the items are scored for frequency (1 = very rarely, 10 = almost always) and eleven of the items are scored for intensity (1 = not much, 10 = a great deal). Subjects were asked to describe their closest relationship along this ten-point rating scale. Items included: "How often do you feel close to him/her? How satisfying is your relationship with him/her? and How much damage is caused by a typical disagreement in your relationship with him/her?" High total scores indicate high levels of intimacy currently being experienced. Internal Consistency, as measured by the Chronbach alpha, is .91 and test-retest reliability is .96

(Miller & Lefcourt, 1982). Concurrent validity has been indicated by significant, positive correlation with high levels of trust and intimacy on the Interpersonal Relationship Scale and significant, negative correlation with loneliness (Miller & Lefcourt, 1982).

Statistical Analyses

Several researchers have indicated that there are many variables affecting children's adjustment to parental divorce that should be statistically controlled (Atkeson, Forehand, & Rickard, 1982; Kanoy & Cunningham, 1984; Lopez, 1987). These variables include parental remarriage, custody agreements, socio-economic status, and religion (Booth et al., 1984; Fine et al., 1983; Gabardi & Rosén, 1991; Lopez, 1987; Santrock, 1987). These covariates are not considered primary variables affecting adjustment to divorce and thus were not chosen as predictor variables in the present study. The predictor variables for the present study were chosen a priori based upon evidence from research indicating the primary importance of gender, marital status, parental marital conflict, and number of years since the divorce in predicting adjustment to parental divorce (Gabardi & Rosén, in press; Kurdek & Siesky, 1980; Rutter, 1970; Wallerstein & Kelly, 1980).

The degree of association between several covariates and the outcome measures was examined. These covariates were mother's remarriage, father's remarriage, with whom the student lived after the divorce, highest level of the parents' education, where the student lives at college, and the student's religion. The covariates that were significantly correlated with outcome measures were entered into simple stepwise regression analyses to determine if each covariate accounted for a significant amount of variance in the outcome variable. See Table 2 for a summary of these results. Residual analyses were conducted to partial out the variance accounted for by the covariates from the respective outcome measures.

RESULTS

Multivariate Analyses of Variance

Separate multivariate analyses were conducted for the sexual behavior measures (total number of sexual partners and the SIS

Table 2

Covariates that were Significant Predictors of Outcome Measures

Covariate	Outcome Measure	R^2	df	F
Mother's remarriage	SIS: Experienced			
	First date	.044	(1,109)	4.99*
	HSE: Morality	.038	(1,109)	4.27*
Father's remarriage	RSE	.072	(1,102)	7.97**
Religion	SIS: Would Like			
	First Date	.050	(1,298)	15.70***
	Several Dates	.016	(1,298)	4.76*
	Total	.058	(1,298)	18.18***
	SIS: Experienced			
	Total	.024	(1,298)	7.24**
Where live at college	Total Number of			
	Sexual Partners	.026	(1,288)	7.63**
	HSE: Morality	.018	(1,288)	5.18**
Parents' education	RBI	.124	(1,282)	40.09***

*$p<.05$, **$p<.01$, ***$p<.001$

scales) and for the belief and attitude measures (Attitudes Toward Marriage, RBI, MSIS, RSE, and HSE). For each of the following multivariate analyses of variance (MANOVA), a Bartlett's test of sphericity and Bartlett Box F were conducted to test the intercorrelation of all outcome measures and homogenelty of variance, respectively. In each case, these tests indicated that all assumptions for the MANOVA were met. Multivariate analyses were based upon N = 263 after subjects with missing data were eliminated from the analyscs.

Sexual Behavior Measures

A 2 X 2 MANOVA was conducted to test the differences among students by parents' marital status (intact, divorced) and the students' gender (male, female) on the sexual behavior measures (total number of sexual partners and the SIS scales). The interaction between parental marital status and gender was not significant.

The MANOVA did reveal a significant main effect of parents' marital status, $F(9,251) = 2.44, p < .01$. Examination of the univariate statistics indicated a significant main effect of parent's marital status on the student's total number of sexual partners, $F(1,259) = 11.27, p < .001$ and on the SIS: Would like (going steady), $F(1,259) = 4.61, p < .05$ (see Figures 1 and 2, respectively). These results show that students from divorced families had significantly more sexual partners ($M = 9.94$, $SD = 15.38$, $n = 94$) than students from intact families ($M = 4.71$, $SD = 6.57$, $n = 166$). In addition, students from divorced families would like to experience more sexual behaviors when going steady ($M = 11.43$, $SD = 1.48$) than students from intact families ($M = 10.85$, $SD = 2.50$). The magnitude of these effects is small (total number of sexual partners omega squared = 0.0379; SIS: Would like, going steady omega squared = 0.0136). Parental marital status accounted for less than 4 percent of the variance in predicting either the student's total number of sexual partners or the number of sexual behaviors a student would like to experience while going steady.

Although not directly pertinent to our hypotheses, the MANOVA

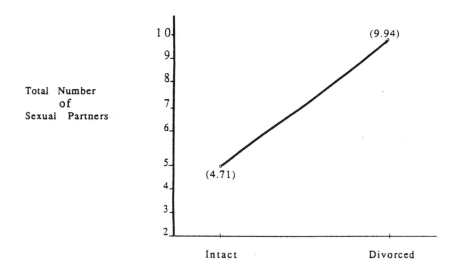

Figure 1. Main effect of parents' marital status on total number of sexual partners.

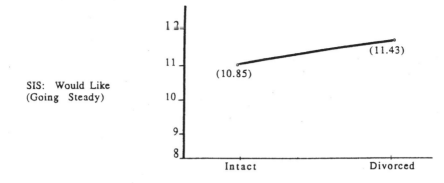

SIS: Would Like
(Going Steady)

Figure 2. Main effect of parents' marital status on SIS: Would Like (Going Steady).

also revealed a significant main effect for gender, $F(9,251) = 8.57$, $p < .001$. Examination of the univariate statistics revealed a significant main effect of the student's gender on total number of sexual partners, SIS: Would like (first date, several dates, and total) and on the SIS: Experienced (first date, several dates, and total). These results indicate that men had significantly more sexual partners than women; $F(1,259) = 15.83$, $p < .05$. Results also indicate that men desire and have experienced a greater number of sexual behaviors on first dates, after several dates, and overall than women; all F's $(1,259) > 6.22$, $p < .05$. The magnitude of these effects is moderate, though variable. Gender accounted for 5.38% of the variance in predicting students' total number of sexual partners (omega squared = 0.0583). Gender accounted for 8 to 18% of the variance in predicting the number of sexual behaviors students would like to experience on a first date, after several dates, or overall (omega squared = 0.0811, omega squared = 0.1790, omega squared = 0.1403, respectively). Gender accounted for 1 to 7% of the variance in predicting the number of sexual behaviors students have experienced on a first date, after several dates, and overall (omega squared = 0.0327, omega squared = 0.0196, omega squared = 0.0668, respectively).

Belief and Attitude Measures

A 2 X 2 MANOVA was conducted to test the differences among students by parental marital status (intact, divorced) and the student's gender (male, female) on the relationship and personal belief attitude measures (attitudes toward marriage, relationship beliefs, intimacy, and self-esteem).

The interaction between parental marital status and gender was not significant, nor was the multivariate main effect of parental marital status. Although not directly pertinent to the hypotheses, the MANOVA revealed a significant multivariate main effect for gender, $F(14,217) = 4.55$, $p < .001$. Examination of the univariate statistics revealed a significant main effect of gender on the MSIS, $F(1,230) = 17.93$, $p < .001$. These results indicate that women experience a higher degree of intimacy ($M = 142.04$, $SD = 16.00$) than men ($M = 132.43$, $SD = 21.09$; $M = 14.37$, $SD = 14.43$, respectively). The magnitude of these effects was moderately low (MSIS omega squared = 0.0544, HSE; Morality omega squared = 0.0667). Gender accounted for 5.44% of the variance in predicting intimacy and 6.77% of the variance in predicting self-perceptions of morality.

MULTIPLE REGRESSION ANALYSES

Three separate series of simple stepwise multiple regression analyses were conducted to determine which predictors (gender, parental marital status, parents' marital conflict, parents' marital happiness, number of years since the divorce occurred, and parental conflict before and after the divorce) were most highly associated with the intimate relationships of college students.

Entire Sample

Simple stepwise regression analyses were conducted to determine which predictors (gender, parental marital status, and parental marital conflict) were most highly associated with the outcome variables (total number of sexual partners, SIS: Would like, SIS: Experienced, Attitudes Toward Marriage, RBI, MSIS, RSE, and HSE). See Table 3 for a summary of the following results. Analyses indicated that gender and parental conflict were both significant predictors of total number of sexual partners. On the first step, gender accounted for 4.88% of the variance, $F(1,224) = 11.49$, $p < .001$ and on the second step, parental conflict accounted for 3.26% of the variance, $F(2,223) = 4.87$, $p < .001$. Gender was a significant predictor on several scales of the SIS: Would like and on two scales of the SIS: Experienced, all F's$(1,224) > 5.63$, all p's < 0.5 (see Table 3). Parents' marital status was also a significant predictor of the SIS: Would like (going steady) scale, $F(1,224) = 4.08$, $p < .05$, accounting for 1.79% of the variance. The direction of these relationships indicate that men have more sexual partners and desire as well as experience more sexual behaviors in dating situations than women. In addition, college students that report their parents having more marital conflict have a greater number of sexual partners. Students from divorced families also desire more sexual behaviors when going steady than students from intact families.

Gender was a significant predictor of the MSIS, $F(1,224) = 9.53$, $p < .005$, accounting for 4.08% of the variance, a significant predictor of the Sexual Perfection scale of the RBI, $F(1,224) = 6.89$, $p < .01$, accounting for 2.98% of the variance and a significant predictor of the disagreement scale of the RBI, $F(1,224) = 4.38$, $p < .05$, accounting for 1.92% of the variance. The direction of these results indicate that women experience greater intimacy in their relationships while men have more idealistic and inaccurate attitudes regarding sexual perfection and avoidance of disagreement in relationships than women. Gender and parents' marital status were significant predictors of scales on the HSE. Parents' marital status was a significant predictor of the Sociability scale of the HSE, $F(1,224) = 4.65$, $p < .05$, accounting for 2.03 of the variance while gender was a significant predictor of the Morality scale of the HSE, $F(1,224) = 9.14$, $p < .005$, accounting for 3.92% of the variance. These findings indicate that students from intact families have more positive self perceptions of their sociability than students from divorced families and women have more positive self perceptions of their morality than men. Finally, parental conflict was a significant

Table 3

Predictors (in R) of Outcome Measures for Students from Divorced and Intact Families

		Predictors	
Outcome Measures	Gender	Parental Marital Status	Conflict
Total Number of			
Sexual Partners	.0488***	---	.0326***
SIS: Would Like			
First Date	.0932***	---	---
Several Dates	.1581***	---	---
Going Steady	---	.0179*	---
Total	.1306***	---	---
SIS: Experienced			
First Date	.0245*	---	---
Several Dates	---	---	---
Going Steady	---	---	---
Total	.0502***		
RBI			
Disagreement	.0192*	---	---
Mindreading	---	---	---
No Change	---	---	---
Sexual Perfection	.0298**	---	---
Sexes are Different	---	---	---
MSIS	.0408**	---	---
RSE	---	---	---
HSE			
Sociability	---	.0203*	---
Morality	---	.0392**	---
Interpersonal			
Relationships	---	---	---
Global	---	---	---
Attitudes Toward Marriage			
Total Score	---	---	.0213*
Doubt	---	---	.0318**
Ideal	---	---	---

*p<.05, **p<.01, ***p<.001

predictor of the Doubt scale of the Attitudes Toward Marriage Survey, $F(1,224) = 7.36$, $p < .01$, accounting for 3.18% of the variance, and of the Total score on the Attitudes Toward Marriage Survey, $F(1,224) = 4.88$, $p < .05$, accounting for 2.13 of the variance. These results indicate that greater parental conflict is related to greater attitudes of doubt and generally more negative attitudes toward marriage. There were no significant predictors of the RSE.

Students from Divorced Families Only

Simple stepwise regression analyses were conducted to determine which variables (gender, number of years since the divorce, parental conflict before the divorce, and parental conflict after the divorce) were most predictive of the outcome variables for students from divorced families. Students from divorced families were analyzed separately to discern if certain factors surrounding the divorce significantly impacted outcome measures. Analyses indicated that gender was a significant predictor of three scales of both the SIS: Would like and SIS: Experienced, all F's$(1,63) > 7.88$ all p's $< .01$. On the second step of the regression analysis, number of years since the divorce was a significant predictor of the SIS: Would like (several dates), $F(2,62) = 10.54$, $p < .001$, accounting for 5.56% of the variance. In addition, parental conflict after the divorce was a significant predictor of the SIS: Experienced (going steady), $F(1,63) = 8.47$, $p < .01$, accounting for 11.85% of the variance. See Table 4 for a summary of these results. These results indicate that men from divorced families desire and experience a greater number of sexual behaviors while dating than women. In addition, more recent parental divorce was associated with greater number of sexual behaviors desired on several dates. Higher parental conflict after the divorce was associated with a greater number of sexual behaviors experienced while going steady. Number of years since the divorce was a significant predictor of three scales of the RBI: the Disagreement scale, $F(1,163) = 5.20$, $p < .05$, accounting for 7.63% of the variance; the Sexual Perfection scale, $F(1,63) = 4.64$, $p < .05$, accounting for 6.87% of the variance; and the total RBI score $F(1,63) = 6.65$, $p < .05$, accounting for 9.55% of the variance (see Table 4). The results indicate that the greater the number of years since the divorce occurred the more negative and unrealistic relationship beliefs in general, and regarding disagreement and sexual perfection. Finally, parental conflict after the divorce was a significant predictor of Attitudes Toward Marriage, $F(1,63) = 4.47$, $p < .05$, accounting for 6.63% of the variance. These results indicate that conflict after the divorce is associated with more negative attitudes toward marriage. Parental conflict before the divorce was not a significant predictor of any of the outcome measures.

Table 4

Predictors (in R) of Outcome Measures for Students from Divorced and Intact Families

Predictors

Outcome Measures	Gender	Years Since Divorce	Conflict Prior	After
Total Number of				
Sexual Partners	---	---	---	---
SIS: Would Like				
First Date	.1111**	---	---	---
Several Dates	.1982***	.0556***	---	---
Going Steady	---	---	---	---
Total	.1558**	---	---	---
SIS: Experienced				
First Date	.1841***	---	---	---
Several Dates	.1853***	---	---	---
Going Steady	---	---	---	.12**
Total	.1959***	---	---	---
RBI				
Disagreement	---	.0763*	---	---
Mindreading	---	---	---	---
No Change	---	---	---	---
Sexual Perfection	---	.0687*	---	---
Sexes are Different	---	---	---	---
Total	---	.0955*	---	---
MSIS	---	---	---	---
RSE	---	---	---	---
HSE				
Sociability	---	---	---	---
Morality	---	---	---	---
Interpersonal				
Relationships	---	---	---	---
Global	---	---	---	---
Attitudes Toward Marriage				
Total Score	---	.0663*	---	---
Doubt	---	---	---	---
Ideal	---	---	---	---

*p<.05, **p<.01, ***p<.001

Students from Intact Families Only

Simple stepwise regression analyses were conducted to determine which variables (gender, parental marital conflict, and student's rating of parents' marital happiness) significantly predicted the outcome variables for students from intact families. Students from intact families were analyzed separately to discover which aspects of intact marriages significantly impacted outcome measures. See Table 5 for a summary of the following results. Analyses indicated that gender and parents' marital happiness were both significant predictors of total number of sexual partners. On the first step, gender accounted for 5.4% of the variance, $F(1,135) = 7.70$, $p < .01$ and on the second step, parents' marital happiness accounted for 3.89% of the variance, $F(2,134) = 6.86, p < .01$. Gender was also a significant predictor of three scales of the SIS: would like. Gender was a significant predictor on this scale for first date, $F(1,135) = 9.01, p < .01$, accounting for 13.31% of the variance and on total behaviors, $F(1,135) = 15.70, p < .001$, accounting for 10.42% of the variance. These results indicate that men have a greater number of sexual partners and desire more sexual behaviors while dating than women. Also, a lower level of parental marital happiness is associated with greater number of sexual partners for college students from intact families.

Gender and parents' marital happiness were significant predictors of several scales of the RBI. Gender was a significant predictor of the Mindreading scale of the RBI, $F(1,135) = 3.97, p < .05$, accounting for 2.85% of the variance and a significant predictor of the Differences between the Sexes scale of the RBI, $F(1,135) = 7.21, p < .01$, accounting for 5.07% of the variance. Parents' marital happiness was a significant predictor of the Partners Cannot Change scale of the RBI, $F(1,135) = 5.96, p < .05$, accounting for 4.23% of the variance. These results indicate that men from intact families have more unrealistic relationship beliefs regarding mindreading and more stereotypic sex role beliefs than women. Also, less parental marital happiness is associated with greater negative relationship beliefs regarding the inability of partners to change. Gender was also a significant predictor of the MSIS, $F(1,135) = 6.15, p < .05$, accounting for 4.36% of the variance and of the Morality scale of the HSE, $F(1,135) = 5.09, p < .05$, accounting for 3.64% of the variance. These results indicate that women from intact families experience greater intimacy and higher self perception regarding morality than men.

Gender and parents' marital happiness were significant predictors of the scales and total score of the Attitude Toward Marriage Survey. Parents' marital happiness was a significant predictor of the

Table 5

Predictors (in R) of Outcome Measures for Students from Intact Families

		Predictors	
Outcome Measures	Gender	Happiness	Conflict
Total Number of			
Sexual Partners	.0540**	.0389**	---
SIS: Would Like			
First Date	.0626**	---	---
Several Dates	.1331***	---	---
Going Steady	---	---	---
Total	.1042***	---	---
SIS: Experienced			
First Date	---	---	---
Several Dates	---	---	---
Going Steady	---	---	---
Total	---	---	---
RBI			
Disagreement	---	---	---
Mindreading	.0285*	---	---
No Change	---	.0423*	---
Sexual Perfection	---	---	---
Sexes are Different	.0507**	---	---
MSIS	.0436*	---	---
RSE	---	---	---
HSE			
Sociability	---	---	---
Morality	.0364*	---	---
Interpersonal			
Relationships	---	---	---
Global	---	---	---
Attitudes Toward Marriage			
Total Score	.0270***	.0764***	---
Doubt	---	.0390*	---
Ideal	---	.0640**	---

*p<.05, **p<.01, ***p<.001

Ideal scale, $F(1,135) = 9.22$, $p < .01$, accounting for 6.40% of the variance; of the Doubt scale, $F(1,135) = 5.49$, $p < .05$, accounting for 3.90% of the variance; and of the total score, $F(1,135) = 11.17$, $p < .001$, accounting for 7.675% of the variance. On the second step, gender was a significant predictor of the total score on the Attitudes Toward Marriage Survey, $F(2,134) = 7.72$, $p < .001$, accounting for 2.70% of the variance. These results indicate that a lower level of parental marital happiness is associated with less idealistic, more doubtful, and generally more negative attitudes toward marriage for students from intact families. Also, men have more negative attitudes toward marriage than women from intact families. Parents' marital conflict was not a significant predictor of any outcome measures for students from intact families.

DISCUSSION

Differences Between Students from Divorced and Intact Families

Sexual Behaviors

The results indicated that college students from divorced families had a greater number of sexual partners than college students from intact families. The results are consistent with research indicating that both male and female college students from divorced families have had more sexual partners (Gabardi & Rosén, 1991; Hepworth, 1984). Other research, however, indicated that only adolescent females respond to parental divorce with increased sexual activity (Hetherington, 1972; Kinnaird & Gerrard, 1986; Lamb, 1977; Sorosky, 1977). Perhaps the inconsistency in these findings is due to the variation in operational definitions and measurement of "sexual activity" or "promiscuity." Also, the differences may be the result of the different age groups studies (i.e., early adolescence, late adolescence, young adulthood). When sexual activity is measured by the total number of sexual partners, this study and others indicate that both men and women from divorced families experience greater sexual activity than their peers from intact families (Gabardi & Rosén, in press; Hepworth et al., 1984).

It may be that college students from divorced families view sexual activity as a means of exploring intimate relationships more than students from intact families. Students from divorced families may have learned from their divorced parents that it is not necessary to be involved in a long-term committed relationship to become sexually involved with someone. Students from divorced families may observe parents having sexual relationships as a means toward finding a more intimate partnership. Sexuality then becomes an important aspect of establishing relationships in efforts to resolve intimacy issues. Another explanation may be that students from divorced families have experienced less parental control and less stringent rules of morality, which may provide more freedom to become sexual with more people (Sorosky, 1977). Finally, some researchers suggest that children of divorce harbor fears of long-term commitment and marriage as a means of establishing intimacy (Despert, 1962; Wallerstein & Kelly, 1987). Perhaps college students from divorced families try to achieve intimacy through sexual activity with several partners, rather than through a committed, emotional relationship with one person.

The results also showed that college students from divorced families would like to experience more sexual involvement (as measured by total number and greater variety of sexual behaviors) while going steady than students from intact families. These results do not indicate what degree of sexual involvement the student had actually experienced, but rather what the student desired to experience. It is interesting to note that there were no significant differences between students from divorced and intact families on behaviors a student would like to experience on a first date or after several dates. There were also no significant differences across groups for sexual behaviors the students have actually experienced. These findings suggest that the differences between the two groups are related to expectations involved within exclusive, committed relationships (defined as "going steady" in this study). Students from divorced families that commit to exclusivity in a relationship desire greater sexual involvement within that relationship. It would seem that, for students from divorced families, the demonstration of increased emotional commitment (via exclusivity in dating) parallels a desire for increased sexual involvement. Students from divorced and intact families do not differ, however, in the sexual involvement that they have experienced.

This finding may indicate that there is a greater discrepancy between what students from divorced families hope for and expect in a "going steady" relationship, and what they actually experience. This could lead to disappointments and dissatisfactions within the relationship; which may relate to findings from previous studies that have indicated that students from divorced families experience less satisfaction, poorer quality, and shorter duration in relationships (Booth et al., 1984; Kelly, 1981). Again, these results showed that both male and female college students from divorced families experience these differences. This result adds further support to the notion that differences in sexual activity for children of divorced parents is not limited to women. No other existing research has directly assessed the differences between sexual activity desired and experienced at various degrees of dating involvement for students from divorced and intact families. This study, however, indicated that students from divorced families may experience a discrepancy in expectation and outcome in more exclusive, committed relationships. This dynamic may have consequences for the student's relationships as commitment increases. Further investigation of this dynamic may prove fruitful in understanding the development of intimate relationships for students from divorced families.

Relationship and Personal Beliefs and Attitudes

The results showed that there were no significant differences between college students from divorced and intact families along these measures (intimacy, relationship beliefs, attitudes toward marriage, and self-esteem). These results suggest that students from divorced and intact families do not differ across attitudinal measures of relationship factors. This result differs from previous studies that have found differences in level of intimacy, relationship satisfaction, fear of commitment, and attitudes toward marriage (Booth et al., 1984; Hillard, 1984; Kelly, 1981). The results, however, are supported by other research that found no differences between students from divorced and intact families in self-esteem and dating satisfaction (Kalter et al., 1985; Kulka & Weingarten, 1979). This result supports the notion that parental marital status is not the most significant factor creating differences among college students along relationship factors. Some studies suggest that the quality of the parents' relationships and the degree of conflict between parents, whether married or divorced, are more salient factors affecting the relationships of college students (Booth et al., 1984; Emery, 1982; Farber et al., 1985; Hetherington, 1979; Raschke & Raschke, 1979). Simply assessing whether college students' parents are married or divorced may not provide enough information on the relationship between parents and/or aspects of the divorce to adequately assess differences across students' relationship beliefs.

GENDER DIFFERENCES

Though not directly related to the hypotheses, it is interesting to note the strength of effects and number of significant differences by gender on sexual behavior and relationship variables. The results showed that men desired and experienced a greater degree of sexual involvement when dating and had a greater number of sexual partners than women. These results indicate that, in general, men desire and experience more sexual activity and diversity in sexual activity than women. These gender differences may be related to sex roles regarding stereotypical perceptions of sexual experience and prowess. For example, in our culture, men receive positive reinforcement for the demonstration of sexual experience and prowess, while women are punished for similar behavior via negative labels ("easy" or "promiscuous"). These social norms may differentially affect the sexual behavior of men and women. Another explanation may involve responding in a socially desirable way on the questionnaire. It may be that the aforementioned sex role stereotypes influence men to exaggerate desired and experienced sexual activity in order to be perceived in the socially desirable "masculine," "virile," or "experienced" way, while leading women to minimize desired and experienced sexual activity in order to be perceived in the socially desirable "feminine," "demure," "chaste virgin" way. These stereotypes may lead women to underreport sexual activity to avoid negative social perceptions.

Results also involved gender differences on intimacy and self-esteem. Women experience a greater degree of intimacy and have more positive self-perceptions of their morality than men. Again, sex-role socialization has given greater permission for women to be more verbal, open, and expressive with feelings than men; all qualities which serve to deepen intimacy in relationships. Also, women have typically taken on the role of caretaker of relationships which gives them more responsibility for creating and maintaining close relationships. It is more difficult to explain the gender difference in self-perception of morality. Perhaps men experience a greater discrepancy between their ideal and real self or between their values and behaviors. Further hypothesizing regarding the meaning of these gender differences is beyond the scope of this study. These findings, however, are interesting and provoke questions regarding the importance of sex roles and gender differences in understanding relationship development in college students.

PREDICTORS OF RELATIONSHIP FACTORS

Students from Divorced and Intact Families

Results showed that the college student's gender and their parents' degree of marital conflict were stronger predictors of total number of sexual partners than parents' marital status (i.e., divorced, intact). Gender was the strongest predictor of total number of sexual partners, consistent with the MANOVA results indicating that men have had a greater number of sexual partners than women. Parental conflict also significantly predicted total number of partners, indicating that greater parental conflict is associated with a greater number of sexual partners. This result is consistent with research indicating that parents' level of marital conflict significantly impacts children, whether parents are married or divorced (Emery, 1982; Farber et al., 1985; Kinnaird & Gerrard, 1986). The results suggest that level of parental conflict is a more significant factor affecting number of sexual partners than parents' marital status. As some studies have indicated, perhaps a more significant question is not whether parents are married or divorced, but how well they get along (Emery, 1982; Kurdek, 1981). It is interesting to note that parental marital status was not a significant predictor when compared to gender and parental conflict, but it did produce significant differences in the MANOVA analysis. One highly tenable explanation is that parental marital status and parental marital conflict are high associated factors.[2] Marital status is a significant factor until parental conflict is considered, at which point conflict becomes a more salient factor. It is quite possible that marital status was not a significant predictor because much of its variance/information was redundant with conflict. This seems likely, given that many divorced couples experienced significant conflict while married (Kinnaird & Gerrard, 1986; Kurdek & Siesky, 1979).

Several other results were consistent with the findings of the MANOVA analyses. Parents' marital status was a significant predictor of the degree of sexual involvement desired while going steady, with both men and women for divorced families desiring greater sexual involvement. Gender was a significant predictor of sexual involvement desired and experienced with men desiring and experiencing greater sexual activity than women. These results were not altered by the presence of parents' marital conflict as a predictor variable.

Similar to the MANOVA, gender was a significant predictor of degree of intimacy and self perception of morality. In addition, gender was a significant predictor of relationship beliefs regarding sexual perfection, indicating, that men have more idealistic and unrealistic beliefs about relationships than women. Interpretation of these findings is beyond the scope of this study. Parents' marital status was a significant predictor of self perception of sociability, indicating that students from divorced families have more negative perceptions of their sociability than students from intact families. An explanation of the absence of this finding in the MANOVA analysis is related to the quantity of dependent measures used in the MANOVA. The large number of dependent measures reduces the power associated with finding significance by increasing the treatment degrees of freedom. This is not a problem within multiple regression analyses, as each dependent measure is analyzed separately. Perhaps then, self perception of sociability was overpowered by other nonsignificant dependent measures when they were all grouped together, but became significant when analyzed separately.

Finally, parental marital conflict was a significant predictor of doubt regarding marital attitudes and of general negative attitudes toward marriage. The results indicated that greater parental conflict is more important than whether parents are married or divorced in predicting college student's attitudes toward marriage. This result differs from studies that indicated students' attitudes toward marriage were impacted by parents' marital status (Gabardi & Rosén, 1991; Glenn & Kramer, 1987; Kalter et al., 1985; Kelly, 1981).

These investigations, however, did not assess the impact of parental conflict on attitudes toward marriage. This study suggests that parental conflict is the more important factor influencing students' attitudes toward marriage. Only one other study has directly assessed the relationship between family conflict and students' attitudes toward marriage, finding that greater family conflict predicted more negative attitudes toward marriage (Kinnaird & Gerrard, 1986).

Students from Divorced Families

The results suggested that parental conflict after the divorce and number of years since the divorce occurred were significant predictors of sexual involvement. In addition, gender again was a significant predictor of sexual involvement with men from divorced families desiring and experiencing more sexual involvement across several dating situations. Fewer number of years since the divorce occurred was associated with greater number of sexual behaviors desired after several dates. Students that experienced their parents' divorce more recently were more eager to become sexually involved after several dates than students that experienced the divorce longer ago. A desire to be more sexually involved in a relationship may be a means of dealing with the divorce, or students may be trying to prove that they do not suffer from the kinds of relationships or lack of relationships that their parents do. This result may be related to a reaction of accelerated courtship activity following parental divorce found in previous studies (Hepworth et al., 1984).

Also, greater degree of parental conflict after the divorce was related to a greater degree of sexual involvement experienced while going steady. Conflict following the divorce may leave students bitter regarding their parents' marriage and determined to create a better relationship for themselves. Students may desire accelerated courtship activities via greater sexual involvement while going steady to create a greater sense of intimacy and belonging. In this way, students may prove their ability to create a viable relationship, unlike their parents, and allay their fears of relationship failure (Booth et al., 1984; Hepworth et al., 1984). Sexual activity within a relationship may also be a means of avoiding conflict (for fear of repeating parental patterns) or it may be a means of trying to establish greater intimacy and support outside of the family, following the loss of parental support by divorce.

Results also showed that number of years since the divorce was also a significant predictor of general relationship beliefs and beliefs regarding disagreement of sexual perfection in relationships. The longer ago parents divorced, students experienced more negative and unrealistic beliefs about relationships, such as "disagreement is wrong and to be avoided" and "sexual perfection is to be expected." There are no other studies that have directly assessed the impact of length of time since the divorce on relationship beliefs. Studies have, however, indicated that college age students that experienced parental divorce in their childhood have higher divorce rates and poor relationship quality (Booth et al., 1984; Kulka & Weingarten, 1979). Perhaps relationship beliefs such as these hinder satisfying relationship development and indicate poor prognosis for the success of those relationships. Another explanation is that students with parents that divorced long ago have had more experience listening to parents' negative beliefs based upon their negative experiences in their marriage. Students may have surmised that disagreement leads to divorce and, therefore, is not a quality of a healthy relationship. Also, some students may have been exposed to parents' complaints about their ex-spouse's inadequate sexual performance. Prolonged exposure to these parental perceptions then would impact students' relationship beliefs. It is interesting to note that these results suggest that negative effects of divorce do not dissipate over time uniformly for all issues and consequences, as some studies have proposed (Hetherington, Cox, & Cox, 1978; Parish & Wigle, 1985). There seem to be different responses to divorce both shortly after the divorce and later, as evidenced by responses of college students. Perhaps it would be more accurate to state that the effects of divorce do not dissipate over time, but rather change relative to relationship factors.

Finally, results showed that greater parental conflict after the divorce was a significant predictor of more negative attitudes toward marriage. This result is consistent with the findings for all students. Parental conflict influences attitudes toward marriage. It is interesting to note that conflict prior to the divorce was not a significant predictor of sexual behaviors or relationship factors while conflict after the divorce was. Perhaps the recency of the conflict after the divorce is more impactful or more threatening because the parents are no longer insulated by marriage. Therefore, if the parents experience great conflict after the marriage has ended, the children may be more likely to have a more severed or conflicted relationship with the noncustodial parent. Conflict and number of years since the divorce are important factors affecting the development of relationships for college students.

Students from Intact Families

The results support the need to determine which qualities of intact parental marriages impact students' intimate relationships. Clearly, factors within parent's intact marriages, not just evidence of parental divorce, impact the relationship development of college students. If researchers are going to consider differences between college students from divorced and intact families in more detail, qualities of both divorced and intact parental relationships need more complete consideration. The results showed that gender and parent's marital happiness were both significant predictors of total number of sexual partners, with gender being more predictive. Consistent with other findings in this study, men have more partners than women. Also, less parental marital happiness is associated with greater number of sexual partners. This result is consistent with the results indicating that students from divorced and intact families that experience greater marital conflict have more sexual partners. It would seem that degree of conflict and happiness between parents is related to college students' sexual activity. It is important to note that measures of marital conflict and happiness are different, but have similar outcomes. One might suggest that a low level of happiness indicates the *absence* of positive/rewarding interactions, while conflict indicates the *presence* of negative/punishing interactions. Both lead young adults to have models of unrewarding parental relationships. As a result, students may have low expectations for emotional satisfaction in relationships and, therefore, meet needs through sexual activity.

Results also showed that less parental marital happiness was associated with greater pessimistic beliefs that partners cannot change and more negative, doubtful, and less idealistic attitudes toward marriage. Students that experience a lack of positive interactions or low levels of happiness between their parents may learn negative beliefs about relationships and marriage through parental example. Low levels of rewarding experiences for parents within their marriage may lead parents to complain to children about their spouse, portraying a negative image of marriage. Therefore, students pick up subtle and obvious messages that unhappy marriages stay that way. Perhaps these students have learned from parents that unhappy marriages are to be tolerated, not changed or broken. This family life may reinforce the belief that partners do not change. Also this may lead college students to have great doubts about entering marriage or about the quality of marriage, negative perceptions of marriage, and low levels of idealism about the institution.

It is interesting to note that parental marital conflict within the intact group alone was not a significant predictor, though parental marital happiness was. It is difficult to find empirical evidence to support or explain this result. Most studies that have examined the impact of parental marriage or divorce on children's adjustment have just considered the role of conflict but not the level of marital happiness (Emery, 1982; Emery & O'Leary, 1984; Markman & Leonard, 1985). Greenberg and Nay (1982), however, did suggest that students from unhappy, intact families had similar attitudes toward marriage as students from divorced families. It seems that variables such as marital happiness or satisfaction are an assessment of more positive aspects of the relationship, whereas the most positive measure of conflict is merely its absence. Therefore, a measure of conflict may not give information on the degree of satisfaction attained in a relationship. Perhaps assessment of conflict alone is adequate for studies of divorced parents. It may be safe to assume that these parents lack the satisfaction necessary to maintain a marriage. In studies where parents remained married, however, it would seem important to assess levels of conflict and happiness. The research in marital therapy would indicate that marital distress is not merely a function of the amount of negative interactions, but also the lack of rewarding/positive interactions (Jacobson & Margolin, 1979). Low levels of happiness within a parents' marriage can also lead to distress between parents, which then affects children. Results of this study indicated that parental happiness within intact marriages is a significant factor affecting college age students' beliefs and attitudes about relationships and, more specifically, marriage.

Finally, results showed that men from intact families have more unrealistic relationship beliefs regarding mindreading and sex role stereotypes, experience less intimacy, and have lower self perceptions of their morality than women. The consistent findings in this study that indicate that gender is significantly related to intimacy and relationship beliefs deserves further study.

CONCLUSION

Establishing intimate relationships is developmentally important to college students. Research suggests that some factors that impact establishing and maintaining intimate relationships include the parents' marital relationship, parental divorce, and factors such as conflict and time following the divorce. Relationship factors that are particularly affected involve number of sexual partners, sexual involvement while dating, relationship beliefs, and attitudes toward marriage. Not only parental divorce, but the quality of intact parental marriages are salient factors affecting the relationships of college students. The intimate relationships of students' parents seems to be a significant part of the process of students resolving their own struggles with intimate relationships.

NOTES

1. Sexual orientation and sexual assault are two factors that significantly influence the development of intimate relationships, these factors could therefore impact outcome factors associated with intimate relationships more than parents' marital status or other predictors. Due to this confound, and in order to create a more homogeneous sample, only heterosexuals with no history of sexual abuse were included in this study.

2. In the present study, parental marital status and parental conflict were significantly correlated, $r = .4314, p < .001$.

REFERENCES

Atkeson, B. M., Forehand, R. L., Rickard, K. M. (1982). The effects of divorce on children. In B. B. Lahey and A. E. Kazdin (Eds.), *Advances in Clinical Child Psychology,* (pp. 225-281). New York: Plenum Press.

Bentler, P. M. (1968). Heterosexual behavior assessment.– I, II. *Behavior Research and Therapy, 6,* 21-30.

Booth, A., Brinkerhoff, D. B., & White, L. K. (1984). The impact of parental divorce on courtship. *Journal of Marriage and the Family, 46,* 85-94.

Cooney, T. M., Smyer, M. S., Hagestad, G. O., & Klock, R. (1986). Parental divorce in young adulthood: Some preliminary findings. *American Journal of Orthopsychiatry, 56,* 470-477.

Eidelson, R. J. & Epstein, N. (1982). Cognition and relationship maladjustment: Development of a measure of dysfunctional relationship beliefs. *Journal of Consulting and Clinical Psychology, 50,* 715-720.

Emery, R. E. (1982). Interparental conflict and the children of discord and divorce. *Psychological Bulletin, 92,* 310-330.

Emery, R. E. & O'Leary, K. D. (1984). Marital discord and child behavior problems in a nonclinic sample. *Journal of Abnormal Child Psychology, 12,* 411-420.

Farber, S. S., Felner, R. D., Primavera, J. (1985). Parental separation/divorce and adolescents: An examination of factors mediating adaptation. *American Journal of Community Psychology, 13,* 171-185.

Farber, S. S., Primavera, J., & Felner, R. D. (1983). Older adolescents and parental divorce: Adjustment problems and mediators of coping. *Journal of Divorce, 7,* 59-75.

Fine, M. A., Moreland, J. R., & Schwebel, A. I. (1983). Long-term effects of divorce on parent-child relationships. *Developmental Psychology, 19,* 703-713.

Gabardi, L. & Rosén, L. A. (1991). Differences between college students from divorced and intact families. *Journal of Divorce & Remarriage, 15,* 175-191.

Glenn, N. D. & Kramer, K. B. (1987) . The marriages and divorces of the children of divorce. *Journal of Marriage and the Family, 49,* 811-825.

Greenberg, E. F. & Nay, W. R. (1982). The intergenerational transmission of marital instability reconsidered. *Journal of Marriage and the Family, 44,* 335-347.

Grossman, S. M., Shea, J. A., & Adams, G. R. (1980). Effects of parental divorce during early childhood on ego development and identity formation of college students. *Journal of Divorce, 3,* 263-272.

Hepworth, J., Ryder, R. G., & Dryer, A. S. (1984). The effects of parental loss on the formation of intimate relationships. *Journal of Marital and Family Therapy, 10,* 73-82.

Hetherington, E. M. (1972). Effects of father absence on personality development in adolescent daughters. *Developmental Psychology, 7,* 313-326.

Hetherington, E. M. (1979). Family interaction and the social, emotional, and cognitive development of children after divorce. In V. C. Vaughn & Brazelton (Eds.), *The family: Setting priorities*, (pp. 71-88). New York: Science and Medicine Publishing Co., Inc.

Hetherington, E. M. (1981). Children and divorce. In R. W. Henderson (Ed.), *Parent-Child Interaction: Theory. research and prospects* (pp. 38-58). New York: Academic Press, Inc.

Hetherington, E. M., Cox, M., & Cox, R. (1978) . The aftermath of divorce. In J. H. Stevens & M. Mathews (Eds.), *Mother-Child Father-Child Relations* (pp. 149-176). Washington, DC: National Association for the Education of Young Children.

Hetherington, E. M., Cox, M., & R. (1979). Play and social interaction in children following divorce. *Journal of Social Issues, 35*, 26-49.

Hillard, J. R. (1984). Reactions of college students to parental divorce. *Psychiatric Annals, 14*, 663-670.

Jacobson, N. S. & Margolin, G. (1979) . *Marital therapy: Strategies based on social learning and behavior exchange principles.* New York: Brunner/Mazel Inc.

Johnson, O. G. (1976). *Tests and Measurements in Child Development: Handbook 11* (Vol, 2, pp. 272-278). San Francisco: Jossey-Bass Inc., Publishers.

Kalter, N., Riember, B., Brickman, A., & Woo Chen, J. (1985). Implications of parental divorce for female development. *Journal of the American Academy of Child Psychiatry, 24*, 538-544.

Kanoy, K. W. & Cunningham, J. L. (1984). Consensus or confusion in research on children and divorce: conceptual and methodological issues. *Journal of Divorce, 7*, 45-71.

Kelly, J. B. (1981). Observations on adolescent relationships five years after divorce. *Adolescent Psychiatry, 9*, 133-141.

Kinnaird, K. L. & Gerrard, M. (1986) . Premarital sexual behavior and attitudes toward marriage and divorce among young women as a function of their mothers' marital status. *Journal of Marriage and the Family, 48*, 757-565.

Kulka, R. A. & Weingarten, H. (1979). The long-term effects of parental divorce in childhood on adult adjustment. *Journal of Social Issues, 35*, 50-77.

Kurdek, L. A. (1981). An integrative perspective on children's divorce adjustment. *American Psychologist, 36*, 856-866.

Kurdek, L. A. & Siesky, A. E., Jr. (1980). The effects of divorce on children: the relationship between parent and child perspective. *Journal of Divorce, 4*, 85-99.

Lamb, M. E. (1977). The effects of divorce on children's personality development. *Journal of Divorce, 1*, 163-174.

Lopez, F. G. (1987). The impact of parental divorce on college student development. *Journal of Counseling and Development, 65*, 484-486.

McCabe, M. P. & Collins, J. K. (1984). Measurement of depth of desired and experienced sexual involvement at different stages of dating. *The Journal of Sex Research, 20*, 377-390.

Markman, H. J. & Leonard, D. J. (1985). Marital discord and children at risk:

Implications for research and prevention. *Early Identification of Children at Risk: An International Perspective* (pp. 59-78). New York: Plenum Press.

Messer, B. J. & Harter, S. (1986). *Manual for the Adult Self-Perception Profile.* Unpublished manuscript.

Miller, R. S. & Lefcourt, H. M. (1982). The assessment of social intimacy. *Journal of Personality Assessment, 46*, 514-518.

Parish, T. S. (1981). The impact of divorce on the family. *Adolescence, 16*, 577-580.

Parish, T. S. & Wigle, S. E. (1985). A longitudinal study of the impact of parental divorce on adolescents' evaluations of self and parents. *Adolescence, 20*, 239-244.

Raschke, H. J. & Raschke, V. J. (1979). Family conflict and children's self-concepts: A comparison of intact and single-parent families. *Journal of Marriage and the Family, 41*, 367-374.

Reiss, I. L. (1967). *The Social Context of Premarital Sexual Permissiveness.* New York: Holt, Rinehart, and Winston.

Rosenberg, M. (1965). *Society and the Adolescent Self Esteem.* Princeton, NJ: Princeton University Press.

Rosenberg, M. (1972). The broken family and self-esteem. In I.L. Reiss (Ed.), *Readings on the Family System* (pp. 518-530). New York: Holt, Rinehart, and Winston, Inc.

Rutter, M. (1971). Parent-child separation: Psychological effects on the children. *Journal of Child Psychology and Psychiatry, 12*, 233-260.

Santrock, J. W. (1987). The effects of divorce on adolescents: Needed research perspectives. *Family Therapy, 14*, 147-159.

Sorosky, A. D. (1977). The psychological effects of divorce on adolescents. *Adolescence, 12*, 123-136.

Vess, J. D., Jr., Schwebel, A. I., & Moreland, J. (1983). The effects of early parental divorce on the sex role development of college students. *Journal of Divorce, 7*, 83-95.

Wallerstein, J. S. (1987). Children of divorce: Report of a ten-year follow-up of early latency-age children. *American Journal of Orthopsychiatry, 57*, 199-211.

Wallerstein, J. S. & Kelly, J. B. (1980). *Surviving the Breakup: How children and parents cope with divorce.* New York, NY: Basic Books, Inc.

Favorable Outcomes in Children
After Parental Divorce

David Gately
Andrew I. Schwebel

SUMMARY. The present paper is based on a review of the literature that considers the short- and long-term effects parental divorce has on children. Most studies in this literature have identified unfavorable outcomes that develop in many areas of children's lives as they struggle to cope with their changed family situations. However, as children adjust to the challenges they face before, during, and after parental divorce, neutral and favorable outcomes are also possible in one or more areas of their lives. In fact, the literature review indicated that many investigators have identified certain strengths in children who had experienced parental divorce. In particular they have observed that following the divorce of their parents some children, in comparison to peers or their own pre-divorce development, have shown enhanced levels of functioning in four areas: maturity, self-esteem, empathy, and androgyny.

Over ten million divorces were granted in the United States during the 1980s (U.S. Bureau of the Census, 1990). The great number of people affected by divorce in the second half of the 20th century stimulated scholarly interest in this area. One topic that received considerable attention is the effects of parental divorce on children, a group affected at a rate of about one million per year since the mid 1970s (U.S. Bureau of Census, 1990).

Findings consistently show that children experience distress during the process of parental separation and divorce and that it is

David Gately was a graduate student, and Andrew I. Schwebel, PhD, is Professor in the Department of Psychology, The Ohio State University, 1885 Neil Ave Mall, Columbus, OH 43210.

© 1992 by The Haworth Press, Inc. All rights reserved.

57

associated with a variety of short- and long-term negative outcomes (see reviews by Anthony, 1974; Fry & Addington, 1985; Kelly, 1988; Kurdek, 1981, Long & Forehand, 1987; Lopez, 1987; San trock, 1987). Wallerstein and Blackeslee (1989) stated, "Almost all children of divorce regard their childhood and adolescence as having taken place in the shadow of divorce. . . . Almost half of the children entered adulthood as worried, underachieving, self-deprecating, and sometimes angry young men and women" (pp. 298-299).

In fact, studies indicate that children may experience difficulties in interpersonal relationships, school behavior, academic achievement, self-esteem, in future life outlook, etc. Besides delineating the wide range of unfavorable outcomes that can develop in children before, during, and after the divorce, the literature also identifies factors that can moderate and exacerbate the problems children face.

Although much of the literature discusses children's struggle to cope with parental divorce and the unfavorable outcomes they may experience in one or more aspects of their lives, some children in adjusting to their changed circumstances before, during, and after parental divorce may also become strengthened in one or more areas. These individuals develop competencies or grow psychologically because of what they learn while undertaking the divorce-related challenges they face and/or because of the changes they experience in self-view as a result of successfully meeting the challenges.

Decades ago Bernstein and Robey (1962) suggested that successful coping with the demands presented by parental divorce can spur emotional and personality growth in children. Since then a number of investigators have found these favorable outcomes in youngsters relative either to their pre-divorce status or to matched peers from intact family backgrounds. (These include: Grossman, Shea, & Adams, 1980; Hetherington, 1989; Kelly & Wallerstein, 1976; Kurdek & Siesky, 1979, 1980a, 1980b, 1980c; MacKinnon, Stoneman & Brody 1984; Reinhard, 1977; Richmond-Abbott, 1984; Rosen, 1977; Santrock & Warshak, 1979; Slater, Stewart, & Linn, 1983; Springer & Wallerstein, 1983; Wallerstein, 1984, 1985a, 1987; Wallerstein & Kelly, 1974, 1976, 1980b; Warshak & Santrock, 1983; Weiss, 1979.)

The present paper is based on a comprehensive review of the literature that investigated post-divorce outcomes in children. The review included literature generated from computer searches of the Psychological Abstracts and Family Resources and Educational Resources Information Center data bases. Manual searches of the Psychological Abstracts, The Inventory of Marriage and Family Literature, and the Social Sciences Index bases were conducted to supplement the computer searches. Finally, empirical and theoretical contributions published in books, chapters, and Dissertation Abstracts were reviewed. Following a brief assessment of this body of literature, the present paper focuses on those studies that reported favorable outcomes in children following parental divorce.

Most of the earliest investigations used a pathogenic model that viewed the divorced family as a deviation from the traditional 2-parent family, and attempted to link this "inferior" family structure to negative effects on children's adjustment and psychosocial development (Levitin, 1979). The picture of the effects of parental divorce on children were further colored in a negative way because these projects typically employed clinical samples and studied the crisis period immediately following divorce (Bernstein & Robey, 1962; Kalter, 1977; McDermott, 1968; Westman, 1972).

Later studies employing non-clinical samples showed that, although divorce is associated with an initial crisis reaction in most children, long-term consequences are variable (Hetherington, Cox, & Cox, 1982; Hetherington, 1989). While longitudinal studies demonstrated that parental divorce may have long-term negative effects on the social, emotional, and cognitive functioning of children (Guidubaldi & Cleminshaw, 1985; Hetherington, Cox, & Cox, 1985), they also showed that children may escape long-term negative outcomes if the crisis of divorce is not compounded by multiple stressors and continued adversity (Hetherington, 1979, 1989; Hetherington et al., 1982, 1985).

The finding that divorce does not necessarily result in long term dysfunction led to a search for individual, family, and environmental factors that moderate children's adjustment. Researchers found the quality of adjustment related to: the child's gender and age at the

time of separation/divorce (Guidubaldi & Perry, 1985; Hetherington et al., 1982, 1985; Kalter & Rembar, 1981; Wallerstein & Kelly,
1980a); the child's temperament, locus of control, interpersonal
knowledge, and level of coping resources (Ankerbrandt, 1986; Hetherington, 1989; Kurdek & Berg, 1983; Kurdek, Blisk, & Siesky,
1981; Kurdek & Siesky, 1980a); the amount of interparental conflict prior to, during, and following separation/divorce (Emery,
1982; Hetherington et al., 1982; Jacobson, 1978; Wallerstein &
Kelly, 1980b); the quality of parent-child relationships (Hess &
Camara, 1979; Hetherington, Cox, & Cox, 1982; Wallerstein &
Kelly, 1980a); the parents' mental and physical health (Guidubaldi
& Cleminshaw, 1985; Guidubaldi & Perry, 1985); the type of custody arrangement (Ambert, 1984; Lowery & Settle, 1985; Santrock &
Warshak, 1979; Santrock, Warshak, & Elliot, 1982; Warshak &
Santrock, 1983; Wolchik, Braver, & Sandler, 1985); parental remarriage (Clingempeel & Segal, 1986; Hetherington et al., 1982; Santrock, Warshak, Lindbergh & Meadows, 1982); the number of major life changes experienced following divorce (Hetherington et al.,
1985; Stolberg, Camplair, Currier, & Wells, 1987), including the
amount of financial decline experienced by the post-divorce family
(Desimone-Luis, O'Mahoney, & Hunt, 1979); and the social support available to both the parents and children (Isaacs & Leon,
1986).

Drawing upon the concept of stress, Wallerstein (1983a) and
Peterson, Leigh, & Day (1984) developed models that could account for the absence of negative outcomes in children. For example, Wallerstein conceived of divorce as an acute social stressor that
had consequences and made unique demands on children (differing
from those associated with stressors like the death of a parent).
Although families experiencing divorce and the loss of a parent
pass through similar transitional stages (Schwebel, Fine, Moreland
& Prindle, 1988), studies comparing the short- and long-term effects on children of separation/divorce and death of a parent support
Wallerstein's contention (Boyd & Parish, 1983; Felner, Stolberg, &
Cowen, 1975; Hetherington, 1972; Mueller & Cooper, 1986; Rozendal, 1983).

Wallerstein (1983a, 1983b) described the sequence of adjustments a child must make: (1) acknowledge the marital disruption,

(2) regain a sense of direction and freedom to pursue customary activities, (3) deal with loss and feelings of rejection, (4) forgive the parents, (5) accept the permanence of divorce and relinquish longings for the restoration of the pre-divorce family, and (6) come to feel comfortable and confident in relationships. The successful completion of these tasks, which allows the child to stay on course developmentally, depends on the child's coping resources and the degree of support available to help in dealing with the stressors. Of course, the divorce process also may include pre-separation distress, family conflict, and compromised parenting which both place children at risk and call for them to make adjustments well before the time when the legal divorce is granted (Block, Block & Gjerde, 1986).

Reports describing protective factors that could mitigate negative outcomes for children following parental divorce complemented findings being described in stress research. More specifically, several authors (Garmezy, 1981, Rutter, 1987; Werner, 1989; Werner & Smith, 1982) found that some children, although exposed to multiple stressors that put them at risk, did not experience negative outcomes. Protective factors diminished the impact of these stressors. Although these investigators studied different stressors, their findings were remarkably similar and suggested that the factors which produce "resilience" in children-at-risk fit into three categories: (1) positive personality dispositions (e.g., active, affectionate, socially responsive, autonomous, flexible, intelligent; possessing self-esteem, an internal locus of control, self-control, and a positive mood); (2) a supportive family environment that encourages coping efforts; and (3) a supportive social environment that reinforces coping efforts and provides positive role models (Garmezy, 1981).

These protective factors reduce the likelihood of negative outcomes by means such as: decreasing exposure to or involvement with risk factors; opening of opportunities for successful task accomplishment and growth; and promoting self-esteem and self-efficacy through secure, supportive personal relationships (Rutter, 1987). Besides helping children avoid short-term harm, these resiliency-building factors strengthen children so they will cope more effectively with and master the stressful life events they will encounter in the future. This "steeling" effect is a favorable outcome that develops after an exposure to stressors of a type and degree that is manageable in the context of the child's capacities and social situation (Rutter, 1987).

The number of studies that identify favorable outcomes of any type for children following parental divorce is small in contrast to the number of studies that have reported unfavorable outcomes. To state the obvious, this difference in the volume of research reports primarily reflects the reality of what children face before, during, and after their parents' divorce. However, a small yet significant part of the difference may be due to the way science has addressed the question of children's outcomes. Specifically, the content of the literature has certainly been shaped, in part, by the fact that neither the pathological nor the stress models heuristically guide researchers to search for favorable outcomes (Kanoy & Cunningham, 1984; McKenry & Price, 1984, 1988; Scanzoni, Polonko, Teachman, & Thompson, 1988) and the fact that the research methods which have been typically employed are more likely to detect negative consequences than positive ones (Blechman, 1982; Kanoy & Cunningham, 1984). For instance, the wide use of measures that identify weaknesses (Blechman, 1982; Kanoy & Cunningham, 1984) and of subjects drawn from clinical samples, who are more maladjusted than their peers (Isaacs, Leon, & Donohue, 1987), makes the likelihood of detecting favorable outcomes unlikely (Kanoy & Cunningham, 1984).

A similar issue is presented by the tendency among researchers to neglect children as a source of data while, at the same time electing to use informants (eg., parents, teachers, clinicians) aware of children's family status (Kanoy & Cunningham, 1984). Although parents' ratings of their elementary school children's adjustment is not related to the children's assessment of the emotional support they are receiving, the children's self-rating of their adjustment are significant (Cowen, Pedro-Carroll & Alpert-Gillis, 1990). Teachers hold more negative expectations for children from divorced families than for their counterparts from intact families (Ball, Newman, & Scheuren, 1984) while parents and clinicians, in contrast to the children, tend to overestimate the negative effects of the divorce (Forehand, Brody, Long, Slotkin, & Fauber, 1986; Wolchik, Sandler, Braver, & Fogas, 1985). In fact, correlations between children's ratings of their own post-divorce adjustment and their parent's ratings are typically low (Kurdek & Siesky, 1980b), a finding consistent with correlations found between children's self-ratings and the ratings of adult informants in other areas of the literature (Achenbach, McConaughy & Howell, 1987).

REPORTS OF FAVORABLE POST-DIVORCE OUTCOMES

Along with the methodologically sound investigations in the divorce literature, there are some studies that have identified favorable post-divorce outcomes in children which suffer from the same weaknesses found in some studies identifying unfavorable post-divorce outcomes: (1) a lack of adequate control for possible confounding variables (e.g., parental conflict, SES), (2) the use of non-representative or inadequately defined samples, (3) the absence of comparison groups of intact families or of subjects matched on relevant variables, (4) measurement problems, including a reliance on informants aware of children's family status, the use of instruments of unknown reliability and validity, and the failure to measure variables that might influence outcomes (e.g., children's social support, temperament, and emotional and cognitive capacities), (5) a tendency to suggest causal relationships from correlational results, and (6) the absence of multivariate interactional models to explain the range of positive and negative outcomes identified. Therefore caution must be used in drawing conclusions from this literature.

The developmental perspective: The research programs of Hetherington and Wallerstein and Kelly and their collaborators show the value of longitudinal work in this area and direct attention to two basic factors: children's developmental level at the time of their parents' separation and divorce and the amount of time that has elapsed between measurement and the point of separation/divorce. The work of each team will be discussed briefly, with attention paid to the areas in which they report favorable outcomes.

Wallerstein and Kelly (1980a) traced the adjustment of an initial sample of 131 children, aged 2½ to 18 years old, from 60 mother-custody families who were offered prevention-oriented psychological assistance. The investigators interviewed the children and family members at separation, 1 year, 5 years, and 10 years post-separation. Although the method used has been strongly criticized, the project merits consideration because it suggests the kinds of favorable out comes that can emerge in the aftermath of parental divorce.

At one year post-separation, Wallerstein and Kelly (1975) identified no positive outcomes among preschoolers (2 to 6 years old). However, a number of early latency age children (7 to 8 years old) had acquired a more realistic view of the world and enhanced self-esteem (Wallerstein & Kelly, 1976). This increase in self-esteem was found only in children who had distanced themselves from parental pressures for allegiance and, in this way, evidently experienced mastery of a difficult situation.

Later latency age (9 to 10 years old) children demonstrated an increased empathy towards one or both parents (Wallerstein & Kelly, 1976), appearing to perceive their parents' needs with great sensitivity. They also provided emotional support to and assumed responsibilities for younger siblings, seemingly benefiting in terms of an enhanced interpersonal knowledge and skill.

Positive outcomes at one year post-separation for adolescents (12 to 18 years) included increases in maturity, independence, self-esteem, and empathy (Springer & Wallerstein, 1983; Wallerstein & Kelly, 1974), as evidenced by mature attitudes toward financial matters (e.g., increased capacity for delay of gratification, more realistic understanding of financial priorities, and gratefulness for what they had), an increased understanding of the need for self-reliance, a more realistic view of their parents' strengths, weaknesses, and personality differences, a more realistic view of the hazards and potentials of marriage, a consolidation of independent moral and ethical standards, and an increased willingness to assume personal and family responsibilities. Gains in self-esteem and empathy appeared to be a function of successful coping with parental pressures for allegiance, an increased sense of competence associated with a marked growth in independence, and an increase in compassion and warmth toward one or both parents.

At five years post-divorce, Wallerstein and Kelly (1980b) reported that 34% of the children possessed high levels of self-esteem and were coping competently at home and school. A number of children at all ages displayed signs of increased maturity, independence, and empathy.

At 10 years post-divorce, maturity and empathy were evident in many children who were preschoolers at the time of divorce (Wallerstein, 1984). They reported appreciating the efforts and sacrifices of their custodial mothers, an increased awareness of financial matters, and a respect for the importance of carefully choosing a marital partner. Many children who were early latency age at the time of divorce spoke proudly of their independence and self-sufficiency (Wallerstein, 1987), and many who had been in their late latency or adolescence reported having a fuller appreciation of the mate-selection task, and an enhanced inner-strength and sense of realism, determination, and responsibility to self and others (Wallerstein, 1985a).

As noted earlier, the confidence in and the generalizability of Wallerstein and Kelly's findings are limited because of the absence of an appropriate intact family control group, the fact that subjects were offered treatment, and the lack of demonstrated reliability and validity of the data-collection methods employed. These difficulties were not found in the project conducted by Hetherington, Cox, and Cox (1982, 1985). They initially studied 144 preschoolers, half of whom were from divorced, mother-custody homes and half (matched on age, sex, birth order, and preschool attended) from never-divorced intact families. Six years later additional data was obtained from 124 of the original families and from new subjects, including children from single-parent mother custody, two parent intact, and remarried stepfather families.

Cluster analyses of adjustment measures at the time of the follow-up indicated that while children who experienced parental divorce were overrepresented in the maladaptive aggressive, insecure cluster (unhappy, lonely, and angry children), they were also overrepresented in the opportunistic-competent and caring-competent clusters, two that involved successful coping (Hetherington, 1989). They were assertive, self-sufficient, high in self-esteem, and popular. Further, they were interpersonally skilled and able in dealing with stressful and demanding situations. The children in these two clusters had adapted well, likely because they had each had a caring adult involved in their lives.

Hetherington (1989) made other observations about the children in each of these two clusters. Almost all children in the caring-competent cluster were girls, half of whom were from divorced mother-headed households. A unique factor in their background was that they assumed responsibility for the care of others at a young age. The children in the opportunistic-competent cluster had a self-centered, manipulative quality to their behavior and frequently came from families in which one parent had personal adjustment problems or neglected or rejected them.

The review of these two projects and of the other studies in the divorce-adjustment literature suggested four areas, in particular, in which children may experience favorable outcomes following their parents' divorce: in maturity, self-esteem, empathy, and androgyny. Each is discussed below.

Maturity

Intact families have an "echelon structure" in which parents form the executive unit. In the single-parent home this structure is replaced by a parent-child partnership that encourages children to assume more self and family responsibility and to participate more fully in important family decisions (Weiss, 1979). Such involvement fosters maturity which is evidenced by increased levels of responsibility, independence, and awareness of adult values and concerns.

Studies employing nonclinical samples have supported Weiss's conclusions. Kurdek and Siesky (1980a) reported that about 80% of the 132 5-19 year-old children they sampled (four years post-separation) believed they had assumed increased responsibilities after the divorce and learned to rely on themselves more. Their parents agreed, with about 75% of the 74 parents sampled rating their children as more mature and independent (Kurdek & Siesky, 1980b). Similar findings were reported by Rosen (1977), who assessed children 6-10 years after parental divorce, and by Reinhard (1977), who surveyed 46 adolescents three years post-divorce.

Children from single-parent families spend more time working in the home and taking care of siblings (Amato, 1987; Bohannon & Erikson, 1978; Hetherington, 1989; Zakariya, 1982). These chores can foster maturity in children, if they are age-appropriate and if the children receive adequate support. The maturity may exhibit itself in the form of an increased level of independence, realism, or identity development (Grossman et al., 1980). Single-parents further foster maturity when they (1) involve children in appropriate decision making and in a healthy range of other responsibilities in the post-divorce family (Bohannon & Erickson, 1978; Devall, Stoneman, & Brody, 1986; Hetherington, 1989; Kurdek & Siesky, 1979, 1980a; Reinhard, 1977; Wallerstein, 1985a; Weiss, 1979; Zakariya, 1982), and (2) allow children appropriate access to feelings that they, the adult caretakers, have as vulnerable individuals who may not always be able to meet the children's needs (Springer & Wallerstein, 1983; Wallerstein & Kelly, 1974).

Finally, a distinction is needed between pseudomaturity, a precocious adoption of adult roles and responsibilities, and maturity, an adaptive development that helps individuals cope more effectively. Pseudomaturity is seen in females from divorced families who display flirtatious and attention-seeking behavior with male interviewers (Hetherington, 1972), who engage in earlier and more frequent sexual activity (Boss, 1987; Hetherington, 1972; Kinnaird & Gerrard, 1986) and who possess a greater likelihood of premarital pregnancy (Boss, 1987) than counterparts from intact families. Pseudomaturity is also found in both males and females from divorced families who engage in earlier and more frequent dating activity (Booth, Brinkerhoff & White, 1984; Hetherington, 1972) and marry earlier (Boss, 1987; Glenn & Kramer, 1987) than peers from intact families.

Self-Esteem

Children may experience increased self-esteem in the aftermath of parental divorce because they cope effectively with changed circumstances, are asked to assume new responsibilities, successfully perform new duties, and so forth. Santrock and Warshak (1979) studied 6-11 year old children, three years after their parents' divorce, and matched youngsters from intact, mother-custody, and father-custody families. Father-custody boys demonstrated higher levels of self-esteem and lower levels of anxiety than intact family boys, while the opposite was true for girls. Slater et al. (1983) studied matched adolescents and found that boys from divorced family backgrounds possessed significantly higher levels of self-esteem than boys from intact and girls from both intact and divorced family backgrounds. Girls from divorced family backgrounds had lower levels of self-esteem than their counterparts from intact families. These results are consistent with Wallerstein and Kelly's (1980a).

One circumstance that appears to foster boys' increased self-esteem in post-divorce families is that they may be more heavily relied upon by custodial parents (most of whom are women) than girls, and as a result may gain a new position of increased responsibility and status. A study of children raised during the Great Depression indicated that older children were strengthened by assuming domestic responsibilities and part-time work (Elder, 1974).

Besides developing as a result of an individual's accomplishments, feelings of self-efficacy may also evolve from vicarious experience, verbal persuasion, and a reduction in the level of fear associated with performing particular behaviors (Bandura, Adams, and Beyer, 1977). Concretely, this suggests that divorcing parents benefit their children by modeling adaptive coping behavior (Kaslow & Hyatt, 1982) and by persuading children to be less fearful and to cope more effectively. Children are most likely to develop hardiness in facing post-divorce challenges if the demands upon them are moderate, if their parents support their efforts to perform new responsibilities, and if family members hold a positive view of divorce-related changes (Maddi & Kobasa, 1984).

Empathy

Some children in divorced and single-parent families show increased concern for the welfare of family members (Kurdek & Siesky, 1980b; Reinhard, 1977; Weiss, 1979). For example, Hetherington (1989) found older girls in divorced families, in contrast to peers, are more often involved in supportive and nurturing teaching, play, and caretaking activities with younger sisters and tend to help and share more frequently. Likewise, about 25% of Rosen's (1977) South African children sample reported they had gained a greater understanding of human emotions as a result of their parent's divorce 6 to 10 years earlier.

Although Wallerstein (1985b) suggested that children's increase in empathy does not extend beyond the parent-child relationship, Hetherington (1989) believes the increased empathy and sensitivity may reflect a more general orientation. The conditions prevalent during children's adjustment may determine the extent to which empathy develops and generalizes. If children are encouraged to provide age-appropriate emotional and practical support to family members, they may be able to extend themselves, gaining an understanding of others' feelings and, in this way, practice and refine their role- and perspective-taking skills. Hetherington and Parke (1979) suggested that more advanced role-taking skills are related to increased altruism, prosocial behavior, communication skills, moral standards, and empathetic understanding.

Androgyny

Necessity, encouragement from others, and the observation of models are among the factors that can lead children to shift away from stereotypical sex-role thinking and behavior and toward androgyny. This shift, in turn, can result in increased cognitive and behavioral flexibility (Bem, 1975; Bem & Lenney, 1976; Bem, Martyna, & Watson, 1976).

MacKinnon et al. (1984) investigated the effects of marital status and maternal employment on sex-role orientations in matched groups of mothers and children between 3 and 6 years old. While employment influenced mother's sex-role views, divorce appeared related to children's sex-role views. These authors suggested that the more androgenous sex-role views of the children in the post-divorce homes may stem from the mothers modeling more generalized sex-role behavior, or from the children assuming more non-traditional responsibilities.

Kurdek & Siesky (1980c) investigated the sex-role self-concepts of divorced single parents and their 10 to 19 year old children, approximately four years post-separation. They found that custodial and noncustodial parents and their children possessed higher levels of self-reported androgyny, when compared to published norms, and that the boys and girls possessed more androgynous sex-role self-concepts than a comparison group of children from intact family backgrounds.

Richmond-Abbott (1984) found that the sex-role attitudes of children, ages 8 to 14, tended to reflect the liberal ones of their divorced, single-parent mothers. However, although the mothers stated that they wanted their children to behave in nontraditional ways, children were encouraged to pursue and tended to prefer sex-stereotyped chores and activities. This fits with the failure of others to find an effect of divorce on preadolescent female's sex-role orientation (Kalter, Riemer, Brickman & Chen, 1985; Hetherington, 1972). Another finding, that the girls in the sample did foresee themselves engaging in nontraditional behaviors and occupations in the future, supports a conclusion that clear post-divorce increases in androgynous attitudes and behaviors may not emerge until children cope with adolescent identity issues.

Stevenson and Black (1988) conducted a meta-analysis of 67 studies that compared the sex-role development of children in father-present and father-absent homes. The applicability of their findings to the present issue are limited, however, by the fact that father absence because of divorce was not treated separately from father absence because of death or other reasons. Nonetheless, some conclusions they drew fit well with points made above. Specifically, father-absent female adolescents and young adults were slightly but consistently less feminine than their father-present peers in measures of traditionally feminine characteristics such as nurturance and expressiveness. Similarly, father-absent preschool boys, compared to their father-present peers, made fewer stereotypically sex-typed choices in picking toys and activities. However, older father-absent boys were more stereotypical than their father-present peers in their overt behavior, particularly in the expression of aggression. This latter difference could be reflecting the fact that in a mother-headed household an older boy may be asked to assume "man-of-the-house" duties.

In conclusion, the literature suggests that increased androgyny in children may develop following divorce if parents model nontraditional attitudes and behaviors or if children, by necessity and/or with parental encouragement, engage in nontraditional activities following divorce. While children in adolescence may struggle with androgenous thoughts, feelings, and behaviors, by their late teens and early twenties many will have worked through the issues. For example, two studies used by Stevenson and Black (1988) showed that college men who had experienced father absence reported fewer stereotypical vocational preferences. Finally, methodology has affected findings: While data collected from parents and teachers suggests that father-absent boys' behavior is more stereotypical than father-present boys', self-report measures indicate the opposite. In this connection, teachers' assessments have differed depending on whether they thought they were rating a child from a divorced or an intact home (Ball et al., 1984; Santrock & Tracy, 1978).

RESEARCH AND TREATMENT IMPLICATIONS

Research is needed to identify a full list of favorable outcomes that can emerge following children's adjustment to parental divorce. Longitudinal studies would be desirable, especially those using matched comparison groups of intact family children while controlling for possible confounding variables, including parental conflict and family SES.

Hurley, Vincent, Ingram, and Riley (1984) categorize interventions designed to cope with unfavorable consequences in children following parental divorce as either therapeutic or preventative. The therapeutic approaches, which include psychodynamic and family systems interventions, focus on treating psychopathology, while the preventative approaches help healthy children avoid significant dysfunction by coping effectively with the normal post-divorce crisis reaction. Preventative interventions take the form of school-based support groups for children (Cantor, 1977; Gwynn & Brantley, 1987; Moore & Sumner, 1985; Pedro Carroll & Cowen, 1985) or school and community-based support groups for parents (Davidoff & Schiller, 1983; Omizo & Omizo, 1987) and families (Magid, 1977; Stolberg & Cullen, 1983). Outcome studies show that parents, children, and group leaders believe support groups decrease distress and dysfunction in children (Cantor, 1977; Freeman, 1984; Gwynn & Brantly, 1987; Magid, 1977; Omizo & Omizo, 1987; Pedro-Carroll & Cowen, 1985). At this point, mental health workers could draw from the literature and design a third type of intervention: ones aimed at promoting favorable outcomes in children who must adjust to their parents' divorce.

REFERENCES

Achenbach, T. M., McConaughy, S. H., & Howell, C. T. (1987). Child/adolescent behavioral and emotional problems: Implications of cross-informant correlations for situational specificity. *Psychological Bulletin, 101*, 213-232.

Amato, P. R. (1987). Family processes in one-parent, stepparent, and intact families: The child's point of view. *Journal of Marriage and the Family, 49*, 327-337.

Ambert, A. M. (1984). Longitudinal changes in childrens' behavior toward custodial parents. *Journal of Marriage and the Family*, (May), 463-467.

Ankenbrandt, M. J. (1986). Learned resourcefulness and other cognitive variables related to divorce adjustment in children. *Dissertation Abstracts International, 47* B, DA8628750, 5045.

Anthony, E. J. (1974). Children at risk from divorce: A review. In E. J. Anthony & C. Koupernik (Eds.), *The child in his family: Children at psychiatric risk* (Vol. 3), 461-478. N. Y.: John Wiley & Sons.

Ball, D. W., Newman, J. M., Scheuren, W. J. (1984). Teachers' generalized expectations of children of divorce. *Psychological Reports, 54*, 347-352.

Bandura, A., Adams, N. E., & Beyer, J. (1977). Cognitive processes mediating behavioral changes. *Journal of Personality and Social Psychology, 35*, 125-139.

Bem, S. L. (1975). Sex-role adaptability: One consequence of psychological androgyny. *Journal of Personality and Social Psychology, 31*, 634-643.

Bem, S. L. & Lenney, E. (1976). Sex typing and the avoidance cross-sex behavior. *Journal of Personality and Social Psychology, 33*, 48-54.

Bem, S. L., Martyna, W., & Watson, C. (1976). Sex typing and androgyny: Further explorations of the expressive domain. *Journal of Personality and Social Psychology, 34*, 1016-1023.

Bernstein, N., & Robey, J. (1962). The detection and management of pediatric difficulties created by divorce. *Pediatrics, 16*, 950-956.

Blechman, E. A. (1982). Are children with one parent at psychiatric risk? A methodological review. *Journal of Marriage and the Family, 44*, 179-195.

Block, J. H., Block, J., & Gjerde, P. F. (1986). The personality of children prior to divorce: A prospective study. *Child Development, 57*, 827-840.

Bohannon, P., & Erickson, R. (1978, Jan.) Stepping in. *Psychology Today, 11*, 53-59.

Booth, A., Brinkerhoff, D. B., White, L. K. (1984). The impact of parental divorce on courtship. *Journal of Marriage and the Family, 46*, 85-94.

Boss, E. R. (1987). The demographic characteristics of children of divorce. *Dissertation Abstracts International, 48 1026A, DA8714900*.

Boyd, D. A. & Parish, T. (1983). An investigation of father loss and college students' androgyny scores. *The Journal of Genetic Psychology, 145*, 279-280.

Cantor, D. W. (1977). School based groups for children of divorce. *Journal of Divorce, 1*, 183-187.

Clingempeel, W. G., & Segal, S. (1986). Stepparent-stepchild relationships and the psychological adjustment of children in stepmother and stepfather families. *Child Development, 57*, 474-484.

Cowen, E., Pedro-Carroll, J., & Alpert-Gillis, L. (1990). Relationships between support and adjustment among children of divorce. *Journal of Child Psychology and Psychiatry 31*, 727-735.

Davidoff, I. F. & Schiller, M. S. (1983). The divorce workshop as crisis intervention: A practical model. *Journal of Divorce, 6*, 25-35.

Desimone-Luis, J., O'Mahoney, K., & Hunt, D. (1979). Children of separation and divorce: Factors influencing adjustment. *Journal of Divorce, 3*, 37-41.

Devall, E., Stoneman, Z., & Brody, G. (1986). The impact of divorce and maternal employment on pre-adolescent children. *Family Relations, 35*, 153-159.

Elder, G. H. (1974). *Children of the great depression.* Chicago: University of Chicago Press.

Emery, R. E. (1982). Interparental conflict and the children of discord and divorce. *Psychological Bulletin, 92*, 310-330.

Felner, R. D., Stolberg, A., & Cowen, E. L. (1975). Crisis events and school mental health referral patterns of young children. *Journal of Consulting and Clinical Psychology, 3*, 305-310.

Forehand, R., Brody, G., Long, N., Slotkin, J., & Fauber, R. (1986). Divorce/divorce potential and interparental conflict: The relationship to early adolescent social and cognitive functioning. *Journal of Adolescent Research, 1*, 389-397.

Freeman, R. (1984). Children in families experiencing separation and divorce: An investigation of the effects of brief intervention. Family Service Association of Metropolitan Toronto (Ontario).

Fry, P. S. & Addington, J. (1985). Perceptions of parent and child adjustment in divorced families. *Clinical Psychology Review, 5*, 141-157.

Garmezy, N. (1981). Children under stress: Perspective on antecedents and correlates of vulnerability and resistance to psychopathology. In A. I. Rabin, J. Arnoff, A. N. Barclay, & R. A. Zucker (Eds.), *Further explorations in personality* (pp. 196-269) N. Y.: Wiley.

Glenn, N. D. & Kramer, K. B. (1987). The marriage and divorce of children of divorce. *Journal of Marriage and the Family, 49*, 811-825.

Grossman, S. M., Shea, J. A. & Adams, G. R. (1980). Effects of parental divorce during early childhood on the ego development and identity formation of college students. *Journal of Divorce, 3,* 263-271.

Guidubaldi, J. & Cleminshaw, H. (1985). Divorce, family health, and child adjustment. *Family Relations, 34,* 35-41.

Guidubaldi, J. & Perry, J. D. (1985). Divorce and mental health sequelae for children: A two-year follow-up of a nationwide sample. *Journal of American Academy of Child Psychiatry, 24* (5), 531-537.

Gwynn, C. A. & Brantley, H. T. (1987). Effects of a divorce group intervention for elementary school children. *Psychology in the Schools, 24,* 161-164.

Hess, R. D. & Camara, K. A. (1979). Post-divorce family relationships as mediating factors in the consequences of divorce for children. *Journal of Social Issues, 35* (4), 79-95.

Hetherington, E. M. (1972). Effects of father absence on personality development in adolescent daughters. *Developmental Psychology, 7,* 313-326.

Hetherington, E. M. (1979). Divorce a child's perspective. *American Psychologist, 34,* 851-858.

Hetherington, E. M. (1989). Coping with family transitions: Winners, losers, and survivors. *Child Development, 60,* 1-14.

Hetherington, E. M., Cox, M., & Cox, R. (1982). Effects of divorce on parents and children. In M. Lamb (Ed.), *Nontraditional families: Parenting and child development* (233-288). Hillsdale, N.J.: Erlbaum.

Hetherington, E. M., Cox, M., & Cox, R. (1985). The long-term effects of divorce and remarriage on the adjustment of children. *Journal of the American Academy of Child Psychiatry, 24* (5), 518-530.

Hetherington, E. M. & Parke, R. D. (1979). *Child psychology: A contemporary viewpoint.* New York: McGraw-Hill Inc.

Hurley, E. C., Vincent, L. T., Ingram, T. L., & Riley, M. T. (1984). Therapeutic interventions for children of divorce. *Family Therapy, 9,* 261-268.

Isaacs, M. B. & Leon, G. (1986). Social networks, divorce, and adjustment: A tale of three generations. *Journal of Divorce, 9,* 1-16.

Isaacs, M. B., Leon, G., & Donohue, A. M. (1987). Who are the "normal" children of divorce? On the need to specify population. *Journal of Divorce, 10,* 107-119.

Jacobson, D. S. (1978). The impact of marital separation/divorce on children: II. Interparental hostility and child adjustment. *Journal of Divorce 2(1),* 3-19.

Kalter, N. (1977). Children of divorce in an outpatient psychiatric population. *American Journal of Orthopsychiatry, 47,* 40-51.

Kalter, N., & Rembar, J. (1981). The significance of a child's age at the time of divorce. *American Journal of Orthopsychiatry, 51,* 85-100.

Kalter, N., Riemer, B., Brickman, A., & Chen, J. W. (1985). Implications of parental divorce for female development. *Journal of the American Academy of Child Psychiatry, 24,* 538-544.

Kanoy, K. W. & Cunningham, J. L. (1984). Consensus or confusion in research on children and divorce: Conceptual and methodological issues. *Journal of Divorce, 74,* 45-71.

Kaslow, F. & Hyatt, R. (1982). Divorce: A potential growth experience for the extended family. *Journal of Divorce, 6,* 115-126.

Kelly, J. B. (1988). Longer-term adjustment in children of divorce: Converging findings and implications for practice. *Journal of Family Psychology, 2,* 119-140.

Kelly, J. B. & Wallerstein, J. S. (1976). The effects of parental divorce: Experiences of the child in early latency. *American Journal of Orthopsychiatry, 46,* 20-32.

Kinnaird, K. L. & Gerrard, M. (1986). Premarital sexual behavior and attitudes toward marriage and divorce amoung young women as a function of their mothers' marital status. *Journal of Marriage and the Family, 48,* 757-765.

Kurdek, L. A. (1981). An integrative perspective on children's divorce adjustment. *American Psychologist, 36,* 856-866.

Kurdek, L. A. & Berg, B. (1983). Correlates of children's adjustment to their parents' divorce. In L. A. Kurdek (Ed.). *Children and Divorce* (pp. 47-60). San Francisco: Jossey-Bass Inc., Publishers.

Kurdek, L. A., Blisk, D., & Siesky, A. E. (1981). Correlates of children's long-term adjustment to their parents divorce. *Developmental Psychology, 17,* 565-579.

Kurdek, L. A. & Siesky, A. E. (1979). An interview study of parents' perceptions of their children's reactions and adjustment to divorce. *Journal of Divorce, 3,* 5-17.

Kurdek, L. A. & Siesky, A. E. (1980a). Children's perceptions of their parents' divorce. *Journal of Divorce, 3,* 339-379.

Kurdek, L. A. & Siesky, A. E. (1980b). Effects of divorce on children: The relationship between parent and child perspectives. *Journal of Divorce, 4,* 85-99.

Kurdek, L. A. & Siesky, A. E. (1980c). Sex-role self-concepts of single divorced parents and their children. *Journal of Divorce, 3,* 249-261.

Levitin, T. E. (1979). Children of divorce. *Journal of Social Issues, 35,* 1-25.

Long, N. & Forehand, R. (1987). The effects of parental divorce and parental conflict on children: An overview. *Developmental and Behavioral Pediatrics, 8,* 292-296.

Lopez, F. G. (1987). The impact of parental divorce on college student development. *Journal of Counseling and Development, 65,* 484-486.

Lowery, C. R. & Settle, S. A. (1985). Effects of divorce on children: Differential impact of custody and visitation patterns. *Family Relations, 34,* 455-463.

MacKinnon, C. E., Stoneman, Z., & Brody, G. H. (1984). The impact of maternal employment and family form on children's sex-role stereotypes and mothers' traditional attitudes. *Journal of Divorce, 8,* 51-60.

Maddi, S. R. & Kobasa, S. C. (1984). *The hardy executive. Health under stress.* Chicago: Dorsey Professional Books.

Magid, K. M. (1977). Children facing divorce: A treatment program. *Personnel and Guidance Journal, 55,* 534-536.

McDermott, J. F. (1968). Parental divorce in early childhood. *American Journal of Psychiatry, 124*, 1424-1432.

McKenry, P. C. & Price, S. J. (1984). The present state of family relations research. *Home Economics Journal, 12*, 381-402.

McKenry, P. C. & Price, S. J. (1988). Research bias in family science: Sentiment over reason. *Family Science Review, 1*, 224-233.

Moore, N. E. & Sumner, M. G. (1985). *Support group for children of divorce: A family life enrichment group model.* Paper presented at Annual Meeting of the National Association of Social Workers, New Orleans.

Mueller, D. & Cooper, P. W. (1986). Children of single parent families: How they fare as young adults. *Family Relations, 35*, 169-176.

Omizo, M. M. & Omizo, S. A. (1987). Effects of parents' divorce group participation on child-rearing attitudes and children's self-concepts. *Journal of Humanistic Education and Development, 25*, 171-179.

Pedro-Carroll, J. L. & Cowen, E. L. (1985). The children of divorce intervention program: An investigation of the efficacy of a school based prevention program. *Journal of Consulting and Clinical Psychology, 53*, 603-611.

Peterson, G., Leigh, G. K., & Day, R. D. (1984). Family stress theory and the impact of divorce on children. *Journal of Divorce, 7*, 1-20.

Reinhard, D. (1977). The reaction of adolescent boys and girls to the divorce of their parents. *Journal of Clinical Child Psychology, 6*, 21-23.

Richmond-Abbott, M. (1984). Sex-role attitudes of mothers and children in divorced, single-parent families. *Journal of Divorce, 8*, 61.

Rosen, R. (1977). Children of divorce: What they feel about access and other aspects of the divorce experience. *Journal of Clinical Child Psychology, 6*, 24-27.

Rozendal, F. G. (1983). Halos vs. stigmas: Long-term effects of parent's death or divorce on college students' concepts of the family. *Adolescence, 18*, 948-955.

Rutter, M. (1987). Psychosocial resilience and protective mechanisms. *American Journal of Orthopsychiatry, 57*, 316-331.

Santrock, J. W. (1987). The effects of divorce on adolescence: Needed Research perspectives. *Family Therapy, 14*, 147-159.

Santrock, J. W. & Tracy, R. L. (1978). Effects of children's family structure status on the development of stereotypes by teachers. *Journal of Educational Psychology, 70*, 754-757.

Santrock, J. W. & Warshak, R. A. (1979). Father custody and social development in boys and girls. *Journal of Social Issues, 35*, 112-125.

Santrock, J. W., Warshak, R. A., & Elliot, G. L. (1982). Social development and parent child interactions in father-custody and stepmother families. In M. Lamb (Ed.), *Nontraditional families: Parenting and child development.* Hillsdale, N. J.: Erlbaum, 289-314.

Santrock, J. W., Warshak, R. A., Lindbergh, C., & Meadows, L. (1982). Children's and parents' observed social behavior in stepfather families. *Child Development, 53*, 472-480.

Scanzoni, J., Polonko, K., Teachman, J. T., & Thompson, L. (1988). *The sexual bond: Rethinking families and close relationships.* Newbury Park, CA: Sage Publications Inc.

Schwebel, A. I., Fine, M., Moreland, J. R., & Prindle, P. (1988). Clinical work with divorced and widowed fathers: The adjusting family model. In P. Bronstein & C. Cowen (Eds.), *Fatherhood today: Men's changing role in the family.* New York: Wiley, 299-319.

Slater, E. J., Stewart, K., & Linn, M. (1983). The effects of family disruption on adolescent males and females. *Adolescence, 18,* 933.

Springer, C. & Wallerstein, J. S. (1983). Young adolescents' responses to their parents' divorce. In L. A. Kurdek (Ed.), *Children and divorce.* San Francisco: Jossey-Bass, 15-27.

Stevenson, M. R. & Black, K. N. (1988). Paternal absence and sex-role development: A meta-analysis. *Child Development, 59,* 795-814.

Stolberg, A., Camplair, C., Currier, K., & Wells, M. (1987). Individual, familial, and environmental determinants of children's post-divorce adjustment and maladjustment. *Journal of Divorce, 11,* 51-70.

Stolberg, A. L. & Cullen, P. M. (1983). Preventive interventions for families of divorce: The divorce adjustment project. *New Directions for Child Development, 19,* 71-81.

U.S. Bureau of the Census (1990). *Statistical abstract of the U.S.: 1990.* Washington, D.C.

Wallerstein, J. (1983a). Children of divorce: Stress and developmental tasks. In N. Garmezy and M. Rutter (Eds.), *Stress, coping, and development.* New York: McGraw-Hill Inc., 265-302.

Wallerstein, J. (1983b). Children of divorce: The psychological tasks of the child. *American Journal of Orthopsychiatry, 53,* 230-243.

Wallerstein, J. (1984). Children of divorce: Preliminary report of a ten-year follow-up of young children. *American Journal of Orthopsychiatry, 54*(3), 444-458.

Wallerstein, J. (1985a). Children of divorce: Preliminary report of a ten-year follow-up of older children and adolescents. *Journal of American Academy of Child Psychiatry, 24*(5), 545-553.

Wallerstein, J. (1985b). The overburdened child: Some long-term consequences of divorce. *Social Work, 30*(2), 116-123.

Wallerstein, J. (1987). Children of divorce: Report of a ten year follow-up of early latency-age children. *American Journal of Orthopsychiatry, 57,* 199-211.

Wallerstein, J. & Blackeslee, S. (1989). *Second chances.* New York: Ticknor & Fields.

Wallerstein, J., & Kelly, J. (1974). The effects of divorce: The adolescent experience. In J. Anthony & C. Koupernik (Eds.), *The child in his family: Children at psychiatric risk* (Vol. 3). N.Y.: Wiley.

Wallerstein, J., & Kelly, J. (1975). The effects of parental divorce: Experiences of the preschool child. *Journal of the American Academy of Child Psychiatry, 14,* 600-616.

Wallerstein, J., & Kelly, J. (1976). The effects of divorce: Experiences of the child in later latency. *American Journal of Orthopsychiatry, 46*(2), 256-269.

Wallerstein, J., & Kelly, J. (1980a). *Surviving the Breakup.* New York: Basic Books Inc.

Wallerstein, J., & Kelly, J. (1980b, Jan.). California's children of divorce. *Psychology Today,* 67-76.

Warshak, R. & Santrock, J. W. (1983). The impact of divorce in father-custody and mother-custody homes: The child's perspective. In L. Kurdek (Ed.), *Children and divorce,* San Francisco: Jossey-Bass Inc., Publishers, 29-45.

Weiss, R. (1979). Growing up a little faster: The experience of growing up in a single-parent household. *Journal of Social Issues, 35*(4), 97-111.

Werner, E. E. (1989). High-risk children in young adulthood: A longitudinal study from birth to 32 years. *American Journal of Orthopsychiatry, 59,* 72-81.

Werner, E. E. & Smith, B. S. (1982). *Vulnerable but invincible: A study of resilient children.* New York: McGraw-Hill Inc.

Westman, J. C. (1972). Effect of divorce on child's personality development. *Medical Aspects of Human Sexuality, 6,* 38-55.

Wolchik, S. A., Braver, S., Sandler, I. (1985). Maternal versus joint custody: Children's postseparation experiences and adjustment. *Journal of Clinical Child Psychology, 14,* 5-10.

Wolchik, S. A., Sandler, I., Braver, S., & Fogas, B. (1985). Events of parental divorce: Stressfulness ratings by children, parents, and clinicians. *American Journal of Community Psychology, 14,* 59-74.

Zakariya, S. B. (1982, Sept.). Another look at the children of divorce: Summary report of school needs of one-parent children. *Principal, 62,* 34-38.

Familial Conflict and Attitudes Toward Marriage: A Psychological Wholeness Perspective

Melanie K. Stone
Roger L. Hutchinson

SUMMARY. The present study examined the relationship between current and past familial conflict, as perceived by college students, and their current attitudes toward marriage. This study also explored the relationship between the family structure in which the students lived (intact vs. divorced) and their current attitudes toward divorce. Contrary to expectations, perceived levels of conflict were not significantly related to attitudes toward marriage, and family structure was not a significant predictor of attitudes toward divorce. Compared to students from intact homes, students from divorced homes reported significantly higher levels of conflict in their homes while growing up. Implications of these findings and limitations and recommendations for future research are discussed.

Divorce is a major disruption of the family unit and often occurs when children are at a young and vulnerable age. Many researchers have questioned how children are affected by this disruption in their families and how it influences them in their own adulthood, particularly in their relationships with others and in their own marriages.

Current literature suggests that it may not be the actual event of

---

Melanie K. Stone, PhD, is affiliated with Health Associates, 9240 N. Meridian St., Suite 292, Indianapolis, IN 46260.

Roger L. Hutchinson, EdD, is on the faculty at Ball State University, Muncie, IN.

This paper was presented at the Midwestern Psychological Association Conference, May 1991.

© 1992 by The Haworth Press, Inc. All rights reserved.

the break-up of the marriage that negatively influences later adjustment in children. Other factors, such as the degree of perceived conflict present in the family and the overall family environment, must be considered when assessing adjustment later in life.

Several studies have examined the effects of family structure on children's development (e.g., Guttmann, 1989; Guttmann & Broudo, 1989; Hutchinson, Valutis, Brown, & White, 1989; Johnson & Hutchinson, 1989). While the results remain somewhat inconclusive, it has become apparent that children from divorced homes do struggle with issues not familiar to children from intact homes, and often they respond in negative ways to the events of divorce.

In past studies, some researchers have viewed divorce as a single, stationary event that may be traumatic for some children. Significance has been placed on the actual physical dissolution of the marriage: a child is adversely affected because of the breaking apart of his/her family. This has been referred to in the literature as the physical wholeness position: problems in adjustment are tied to the loss of the parent in the family system (Bach, 1946; Sears, Pintler, & Sears, 1946).

Other researchers tend to see divorce as a process rather than an event. The divorce experience has been extended backward temporally to include the tension and conflict that are often a part of the predivorce experience. This approach has been referred to in the literature as the psychological wholeness position: problems in adjustment are not tied directly to the loss of the parent but rather to the conflict that is often so much a part of the divorce process (Emery, 1982; Kelly & Berg, 1978; Maskin & Brookins, 1974; Nye, 1957).

Recent research has been conducted in an effort to examine more closely the physical and psychological wholeness positions (Dancy & Handal, 1980, 1984; Enos & Handal, 1986). The level of perceived conflict in the family has been found to be significantly related to the adolescent's perceptions of family climate, psychological adjustment, and peer relationships. Dancy and Handal's (1984) research examined the psychological wholeness position. They concluded that "divorce would be better conceptualized as a crisis situation, loss of a two-parent family system, rather than as a uniformly and universally negative event . . . "(p. 228).

These research findings suggest that divorce itself may or may not be a negative event, depending on the degree of perceived family conflict. Adjustment appears to be related to the level of current perceived conflict in the home, rather than to the actual dissolution of the marriage. For some adolescents, finally being free of the conflict-ridden environment their parents have created may result in better adjustment. Still of concern, however, are the effects of being in the conflict-ridden environment for an extended period of time.

Several studies have examined the effects of family structure (i.e., divorced, intact, remarried) on the marital attitudes of adolescents (Amato, 1988; Ganong, Coleman, & Brown, 1981; Robson, 1982). In general, they found there to be no significant differences among adolescents from each of the three family structures regarding their attitudes toward marriage. These findings lend support to the psychological wholeness position.

In addition to research on attitudes toward marriage, researchers have investigated attitudes toward divorce (Coleman & Ganong, 1984; Ganong, Coleman & Brown, 1981; Greenberg & Nay, 1982; Kinnaird & Gerrard, 1986; Rozendal, 1983). Much of the research indicates that children from separated/divorced homes have more favorable attitudes toward divorce than those from intact homes. It seems that being exposed to the event of divorce somehow results in a more favorable attitude toward divorce for the children who observe the process occurring. Greenberg and Nay (1982) suggested a disinhibitory effect of parental divorce on children's attitudes toward divorce.

The statistics on divorce in this country are staggering. As a result, researchers as well as parents, teachers, and other educators are concerned about children who are faced with growing up in these potentially stressful environments. The present study examines the effects of college students' perceptions of family conflict, both past and present, and its relationship to their attitudes toward marriage. It also examines the effects of family structure on students' attitudes toward divorce. This finding would support the psychological wholeness position, thereby removing the negative label from the event of divorce and instead placing the responsibility on the quality of the family environment.

It was hypothesized that there would be a negative relationship between conflict in the family as perceived by students and their attitudes toward marriage, regardless of whether their parents were divorced or intact. It was also hypothesized that students who experienced parental divorce would have more favorable attitudes toward divorce than students from intact homes, regardless of perceived conflict in the family.

METHOD

Participants

Participants in this study were 204 undergraduate students attending a midwestern State University. There were 144 women and 60 men. The average age of the students was 20.7 years, with an age range of 18 to 32 years. All of the students were single; none of the students previously had been married or divorced.

Instrumentation

Three scales were used: (1) The Attitudes Toward Marriage scale, (2) The Attitudes Toward Divorce scale, and the (3) Family Environment Scale (FES).

The Attitudes Toward Marriage Scale. The Attitudes Toward Marriage scale is a self-report questionnaire that was originally published by Wallin (1954) and later revised by Kinnaird and Gerrard (1986). The revised version was used in this study; it consists of 14 items to be answered, using a 5-point Likert scale. The items are comprised of questions such as "If you marry, how happy do you think you will be?" and statements such as "A bad marriage is better than no marriage at all." These questions and statements are designed to assess the subjects' expectations and desires regarding their future marital status. Higher scores indicate more favorable attitudes toward marriage; lower scores indicate more unfavorable attitudes. Past analysis of this scale yielded a Cronbach alpha for internal consistency of .88. The Pearson correlation for test-retest reliability was .87 (Kinnaird & Gerrard, 1986). This instrument demonstrated discriminant validity for its ability to assess marital attitudes by differentiating among intact and father-absent groups on this variable (Kinnaird & Gerrard, 1986).

The Attitudes Toward Divorce Scale. The Attitudes Toward Divorce Scale is a self-report questionnaire based on a questionnaire described by Hardy (1957) and later designed by Kinnaird and Gerrard (1986) in their study of attitudes toward divorce. The revised measure used in this study consists of 12 5-point Likert scale items. Subjects are asked to rate their agreement with favorable and unfavorable statements about divorce (e.g., "Even if people are unhappy with their marriage, they should stay together and try to improve it;" "People should feel no great obligation to remain married if they are not satisfied"). These statements are designed to assess the subjects' expectations and beliefs regarding divorce. Higher scores indicate more favorable attitudes and lower scores more unfavorable attitudes. Past analysis of this scale yielded a Cronbach alpha for internal consistency of .77. The Pearson correlation for test-retest reliability was .86 (Kinnaird & Gerrard, 1986). This instrument demonstrated discriminant validity by differentiating among reconstituted (remarried) families and intact families on attitudes toward divorce (Kinnaird & Gerrard, 1986).

The Family Environment Scale (FES). The Family Environment Scale (FES) is a self-report questionnaire designed by Moos (1974a). It consists of 90 true-false statements that assess the social climate of the family (e.g., "Family members often criticize each other;" "We really get along well with each other"). Of particular interest in this study was the Conflict subscale, which was used to measure the amount of discord subjects perceived in their homes currently as well as while they were growing up. Students were asked to complete the FES two times: (1) They first responded to the statements as they currently applied to their family. (2) They then responded to the statements as they applied to their family while growing up.

Demographic Questionnaire. In addition to the scales, the students were asked to complete a demographic questionnaire. This questionnaire addressed such variables as the student's marital status, the person(s) the student lived with when visiting or staying with his or her family, the time period in which the student lived with the family, the current marital status of the student's biological parents, the level of education completed by the student's parents, and the attitude of the student's religion toward divorce.

Procedures

Questionnaires were administered in a group setting. Participants remained anonymous by not signing their names to any of the materials. Students were given the following testing materials (one at a time): the Family Environment Scale with a focus on current perceptions of family; the Attitudes Toward Marriage scale; the Attitudes Toward Divorce scale; the Family Environment Scale with a focus on past perceptions of family; and the demographic questionnaire. Instructions were given for the scales and questionnaire, and questions were answered concerning the procedure. Testing time was approximately one hour. Following administration of the instruments, participants were debriefed, and the purpose of the research study was discussed.

RESULTS

Description of the Sample

Sample Size. A total of 210 students participated in the study. Five sets of data were eliminated as a result of the students themselves being divorced; only students who had never been married before were included in the study. One set of data was eliminated as a result of incomplete information. This resulted in 204 completed sets of data for analysis.

Sixty-nine percent of the students responded that their parents were currently married to each other. Twenty-five percent of the students reported that their parents were currently divorced from each other. The remaining 6% reported that one or both parents were deceased.

Results of Multiple Regression Analyses

It was proposed that the level of conflict in the family, as perceived by the student both currently and in the past, would account for a significant proportion of variance in scores on the Attitudes Toward Marriage scale. Specifically, the higher the level of conflict, the less favorable the students' attitude toward marriage would be. Hierarchical regression analysis was used, consisting of four predictor variables in four stages. The first step to be entered for each analysis was the block of variables that was addressed on the demographic sheet (religion, sex, education of father, the time period in which the student lived with the family, grade, the parent(s) the student lived with, education of mother, and age). Within the block, these variables were entered in stepwise form. The remaining steps were entered hierarchically.

None of the resulting multiple correlations were statistically significant. Thus, conflict was not useful in explaining variance on the Attitudes Toward Marriage scale; family structure was not useful in explaining variance on the Attitudes Toward Divorce scale.

Results of Unhypothesized Analyses

A *t*-test was conducted to examine the differences between students who came from intact and divorced homes and their attitudes toward marriage and divorce, as reflected on the Attitudes Toward Marriage scale and the Attitudes Toward Divorce scale. There were no statistically significant differences between the groups in either their attitudes toward marriage or their attitudes toward divorce.

A second *t*-test was conducted to examine the relationship between family structure and the Conflict score on the current and past FES. Students in divorced homes ($M = 4.98$, SD = 2.55) scored statistically significantly higher (t [190] = -1.98, $p = .049$) on the past Conflict subscale than students from intact homes ($M = 4.13$, SD = 2.67). Thus, students from divorced homes reported higher levels of conflict in their families while growing up as compared to students from intact homes. There were no statistically significant differences between the current Conflict score and family structure (see Figure 1).

A cross-tabulation was generated for the variables pertaining to parental marital status and the students' self-report of their religion's beliefs about divorce (see Figure 2).

Seventy-two percent of students from intact homes reported that

FIGURE 1

Family Structure and Past Conflict

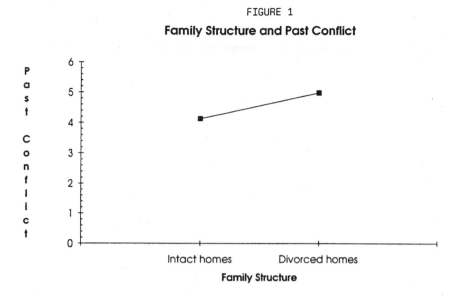

FIGURE 2

Perceptions of Religion's Attitude Toward Divorce

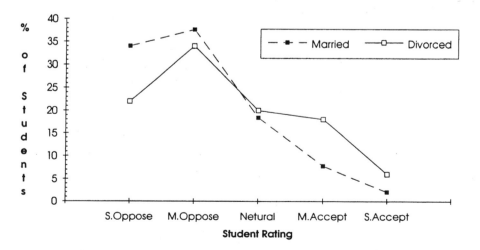

their religion was either moderately or strongly opposed to divorce. Fifty-six percent of students from divorced homes reported that their religion was either moderately or strongly opposed to divorce. Only 10% of students from intact homes reported that their religion was either moderately or strongly accepting toward divorce, while 24% of students from divorced homes reported that their religion was either moderately or strongly accepting toward divorce. The Chi-Square statistic generated for these numbers was not statistically significant.

DISCUSSION

In this study the level of conflict in the home, as perceived by the student, did not significantly predict subsequent attitudes toward marriage. Neither current nor past conflict was useful in explaining the variance on the Attitude Toward Marriage scale. This finding could support the notion that high levels of conflict do not necessarily lead to less favorable attitudes toward marriage. Children may have a certain amount of resiliency when exposed to conflict and may not be as affected in their attitudes toward marriage as one might expect.

Contrary to expectations, family structure was not useful in explaining variance on the Attitudes Toward Divorce scale. Students who experienced parental divorce did not demonstrate a more favorable attitude toward divorce than those students who did not experience parental divorce. This is an area that remains unclear in terms of the influence divorce may have on children's later attitudes toward divorce. Perhaps the findings in Amato's (1988) study reflect more accurately what actually occurs in these children. Amato (1988) found that respondents from divorced families were, overall, more positive than negative in their recollections. This interpretation is consistent with the notion that once family members have time to adjust, family relationships in most one-parent and stepparent families are close and mutually supportive (Amato, 1987a, 1987b; Weiss, 1979). Perhaps more noteworthy in his study is the fact that adult children of divorce were no more or less likely than other respondents to be in favor of divorce. These findings indicate that adult children of divorce are not in any sense pro-divorce or anti-marriage. Instead, the great majority appear to value family life to the same extent that other young people do (Amato, 1988).

No statistically significant differences were found to exist between students who came from intact and divorced homes and their attitudes toward marriage and divorce. According to the hypotheses of this study, no differences were expected to exist for attitudes toward marriage based on family structure; rather, the level of conflict was expected to be the variable that would predict attitudes toward marriage. Differences were expected to exist for attitudes toward divorce based on family structure.

Students from divorced homes scored significantly higher on the past conflict scale than students from intact homes. This finding suggests that those students who grew up in divorced homes perceived more conflict in their families than did those students who grew up in intact homes. This finding makes intuitive sense in that divorce often is accompanied by tension and strife, even after one parent has moved away from the home. At this time, however, no conclusions can be made about the effects this conflict may have on a child's later adjustment.

Some interesting findings were observed when each student was asked to report how his or her religion viewed divorce. Students from intact homes in general reported that their religion was fairly opposed to divorce, while students from divorced homes in general reported that their religion was more accepting toward divorce. This is interesting in that students were asked for their perception of how their religion viewed divorce. It is possible that students who experienced parental divorce altered their view of their religion, making it seem more open toward divorce than it actually may have been.

CONCLUSIONS

The primary intention of this study was to examine the effects of conflict and family structure on attitudes toward marriage and divorce. The results do not, in general, support those reported in the research literature.

It is important to address some of the potential limitations of this study. The FES was used in an attempt to obtain an overall measure of conflict in the home. Since there were only 10 items that made up the conflict subscale, it may have not been a thorough enough or sensitive enough scale. The attitude scales as well may not have been sensitive enough to measure attitudes in a useful way.

Because participants were asked to report on events that occurred in the past, participants may have either forgotten or redefined their family environment as being more or less conflictual than it really was. One could argue, however, that it is the perception on the part of the student that is really important, more so even than how the environment really was. Another possibility is that, if, by adulthood, there are no differences in attitudes, then divorce loses its impact. This would explain some of the continuing preferences for marriage in a society full of divorce.

Conflict in the family would seem to be a negative event for the children involved. Children growing up in a home filled with tension and strife are inevitably affected by such turmoil, perhaps in very different ways. In order for a child to grow up healthily, both physically and emotionally, it is best that he or she experience a positive, nurturing environment.

Determining how familial conflict and dissolution affects the adjustment of college-age students is central to understanding the potentially deleterious nature of this home environment, and ultimately, to the development of treatment and prevention methods to overcome these effects. Unfortunately, not many clear conclusions can be drawn from the present study. The question still remains as to how and in what way students are affected by conflict in their families currently and while growing up. It is not a question of whether they are affected but in what way they are affected. This research has not been able to definitively answer this question. One conclusion, however, might be that conflict does not affect a student's attitude toward marriage in any measurable way. If so, this can be seen as a positive outcome. Consequently, it could be stated that conflict in the family does not seem to result in a more unfavorable attitude toward marriage.

Intuitively, it would seem that family structure and conflict are interacting variables associated with long-term adjustment. To date, the research in this area has been largely atheoretical. Continuing to explore this relationship empirically and integrating findings with theory will facilitate the development of a more complete understanding of the effects of family structure and perceived family conflict. Such an understanding should have therapeutic implications for both the children living in the conflictual environment and their parents who seek counseling for relationship difficulties.

REFERENCES

Amato, P. (1988). Parental divorce and attitudes toward marriage and family life. *Journal of Marriage and the Family, 50*, 453-461.

Amato, P. (1987a). *Children in Australian families: The growth of competence.* Sydney, New South Wales: Prentice-Hall of Australia.

Amato, P. (1987b). Family processes in one-parent, stepparent, and intact families: The child's point of view. *Journal of Marriage and the Family, 49*, 327-337.

Bach, G. (1946). Father-fantasies and father-typing in father separated children. *Child Development, 17*, 63-80.

Bowlby, J. (1973). *Attachment and Loss: II. Separation.* New York: Basic Books Inc.

Coleman, M., & Ganong, L. (1984). Effect of family structure on family attitudes and expectations. *Family Relations, 33*, 425-432.

Dancy, B., & Handal, P. (1984). Perceived family conflict, psychological adjustment, and peer relationships of Black adolescents: A function of parental marital status or perceived family conflict? *Journal of Community Psychology, 12*, 222-229.

Dancy, B., & Handal, P. (1980). Perceived family climate of Black adolescents: A function of parental marital status or perceived conflict? *Journal of Community Psychology, 8*, 208-214.

Emery, R. (1982). Interpersonal conflict and children of discord and divorce. *Psychological Bulletin, 92*, 310-330.

Enos, D., & Handal, P. (1986). The relation of parental marital status and perceived family conflict to adjustment in White adolescents. *Journal of Consulting and Clinical Psychology, 54*, 820-824.

Ganong, L., Coleman, M., & Brown, G. (1981). Effect of family structure on marital attitudes of adolescents. *Adolescence, 62*, 281-288.

Greenberg, E., & Nay, R. (1982). The intergenerational transmission of marital instability reconsidered. *Journal of Marriage and the Family, 44*, 335-347.

Guttmann, J. (1989). Intimacy in young adult males' relationships as a function of divorced and non-divorced family of origin. *Journal of Divorce, 12*, 253-261.

Guttmann, J., & Broudo, M. (1989). The effect of children's family type on teachers' stereotypes. *Journal of Divorce, 12*, 315-328.

Hardy, K. (1957). Determinants of conformity and attitude change. *Journal of Abnormal and Social Psychology, 54,* 289-294.

Hutchinson, R.L., Valutis, W.E., Brown, D.T. & White, I.S. (1989). The effects of family structure on institutionalized children's self-concepts. *Adolescence, 24,* 303-310.

Johnson, M.K., & Hutchinson, R.L. (1989). The effects of family structure on children's self-concepts. *Journal of Divorce, 12,* 129-138.

Kelly, J., & Berg, B. (1978). Measuring children's reactions to divorce. *Journal of Clinical Psychology, 34,* 215-221.

Kinnaird, K., & Gerrard M. (1986). Premarital sexual behavior and attitudes toward marriage and divorce among young women as a function of their mothers' marital status. *Journal of Marriage and the Family, 48,* 757-765.

Maskin, M., & Brookins, E. (1974). The effects of parental composition on recidivism rates in delinquent girls. *Journal of Clinical Psychology, 30,* 341-342.

Moos, R. (1974a). *The Social Climate Scales: An overview.* Consulting Psychologists Press, Inc., Palo Alto, Calif.

Nye, I. (1957). Child adjustment in broken and in unhappy homes. *Marriage and Family Living, 19,* 356-361.

Robson, B. (1982). And they lived happily ever after: Marriage concepts of older adolescents. *Canadian Journal of Psychiatry, 28,* 646-649.

Rozendal, F. (1983). Halos vs. stigmas: Long-term effects of parent's death or divorce on college students' concepts of the family. *Adolescence, 18,* 947-955.

Sears, R., Pintler, M., & Sears, P. (1946). Effects of father separation on preschool children's doll play aggression. *Child Development, 17,* 219-243.

Wallin, P. (1954). Marital happiness of parents and their children's attitude toward marriage. *American Sociological Review, 19,* 20-23.

Weiss, R. (1979). *Going it alone. The family life and social situation of the single parent.* New York: Basic Books Inc.

Differences in the Marriage Role Expectations of College Students from Intact and Divorced Families

Joseph A. Marlar
Keith W. Jacobs

SUMMARY. The differences in marriage role expectations between college students of divorced and intact families were investigated using the Marriage Role Expectation Inventory (MREI). The MREI (Dunn and DeBonis, 1979) measures desires for traditional versus companionship style of marital relationships. It was hypothesized that those participants from divorced families would expect a more companionship oriented marriage role while those from intact families would expect a more traditional marriage role. Participants included 100 male and female students enrolled in introductory courses at Loyola University in New Orleans. Significant gender by marital status interactions were found in total MREI scores, as well as all eight MREI subscores. Males with married parents were more companionship oriented than males with divorced parents. On the other hand, females with divorced parents were more companionship oriented, while females with married parents were more traditional oriented in their marriage role expectations.

The role of the family cannot be overestimated. The family is the environment where the children learn to develop their own ideas of

Joseph A. Marlar, BA, is a graduate student and Keith W. Jacobs, PhD, is on the faculty of the Department of Psychology at Loyola University, New Orleans, LA 70118.

Requests for reprints may be addressed to: K.W. Jacobs, Box 194, Loyola University, New Orleans, LA 70118.

© 1992 by The Haworth Press, Inc. All rights reserved.

what families should be. The style of parenting, system of values, and relationship with loved ones are all taught in the family setting. If this structure is not maintained because of divorce, separation, or death, it is likely to affect the concept that the children of that family hold about their own future marriage and family relations.

Evidence from a ten year follow-up study found that divorce indeed affects adult children's relationships. Wallerstein (1987) reported that separation from families and transition into young adulthood were burdened by fear of disappointment in love relationships, lowered expectations, and a sense of powerlessness by those who experienced divorce or separation in the home. It is suggested that children from divorced and separated families who experienced these difficult transitions may react differently to marriage in the future.

Marriage role expectations are formed throughout the child's life, of which the divorce may be a part. Dunn suggests that "marriage adjustment may be regarded as a process in which marriage partners attempt to reenact relational systems" (Dunn, 1960, p. 99). These reenactments may be traditional or companionship in nature.

Greenburg and Nay (1982) reported a national survey that revealed that children from marriages that were disrupted during their childhood have a higher rate of divorce than children from intact marriages. This higher rate of divorce is coupled with the divorced group espousing the most favorable attitude toward divorce. They also found that, contrary to previous research, there was no meaningful effect of age at time of marital disruption. The fact that these children from divorced parents are more likely to divorce indicates that their attitudes of marriage are somewhat different from those of children from intact families. These differences could also be attributed to gender discrepancies rather than a genuine difference between the two groups of children.

Mueller and Pope (1977) examined the intergenerational transmission of marital instability. They concluded that respondents from parental homes that were disrupted by death or divorce during their childhood had higher rates of divorce or separation in their own first marriages. Therefore, children from divorced families are becoming involved more often in divorce in the next generation than children from families that have remained intact.

Long (1987) conducted a longitudinal study of college females to test the hypotheses that perceptions of parental discord and parental separation would have negative effects on attitudes toward marriage and on courtship progress. These hypotheses were supported by data from 134 female undergraduates who were tested as entering first-year students and again eighteen months later. Daughters of divorced parents married younger, were less well educated, and married men with less desirable jobs. On the other hand the daughters of happy, intact marriages were significantly more positive about marriage and were progressing toward it.

Ganong, Coleman, and Brown (1981) utilized several instruments to measure the marriage role expectations of males and females in an effort to identify gender differences. Female subjects held more favorable attitudes toward marriage and were more egalitarian in their marriage role expectations than were males. There were no sex differences in attitudes toward divorce. This suggests that this susceptibility of divorce among the children from the divorced parents is a function of their parent's marital status.

Carson and Kelly (1990) studied 94 undergraduates who either did or did not have history of parental divorce within the first 18 years of life. Using The Marriage Role Expectation Inventory (Dunn and DeBonis, 1979), they found significant group differences in only 3 measures investigated: sexual relations in marriage, social participation of marriage partners, and the degree of control exhibited in the family. For both social participation and sexual relations, the young adults of non-divorced parents had a lower score than the young adults of divorced parents. The young adults of divorced parents perceived less control and less adaptability in their ideal marriage and family environments. Children from divorced parents were more oriented towards companionship relationships than were the adults from intact parents.

Additional findings are submitted by Kelly (1981) in a study of eighteen 17 to 23 year olds in a five year follow-up study. The children from the divorced families experienced interference with the establishment of enduring ties and formed impoverished, immature, and ungratifying relationships. In addition to this, the study revealed that a very negative view of marriage remained among those who came from divorced families.

A longitudinal study by Weeks, O'Neal, and Botkin (1987) compared the marriage role expectations of 326 female college students in 1961, 1972, and 1978. The group was significantly more egalitarian in overall marriage role expectation in 1972 than in 1961. This trend continued through 1978 but at a slower rate.

The general impact of divorce on the children also reaches into their sexual behavior. Kinnaird and Garrard (1986) examined the premarital sexual activity of 90 unmarried female undergraduates. Subjects from divorced or reconstituted families reported more sexual experience than did those from intact families.

Gabardi and Rosén (1991) support these conclusions with a similar population of 500 college students. Their research found that a significantly higher number of female students from divorced families had engaged in sexual intercourse, and both male and female students had more negative views of marriage than students from intact families. These authors leave questions unanswered regarding how this population expect to function in their own marriages.

Research exclusively with women reports similar findings. Southworth and Schwartz (1987) found that parental divorce had long-term effects on the subjects' expectations about their futures in relation to men, work, and marriage. They tested for the possibility that a difference might be attributable to the relationship that these women had with their father. In the final analysis, these effects seem to be related to the family structure and not a result of the relationship that these women had with their fathers.

The research suggests that parental divorce affects the children's sexual behavior, time of marriage and attitudes toward marriage. From the previous research conducted in this area, it was hypothesized that young adults from divorced families will seek a more companionship oriented marriage style while those from non-divorced families will expect a more traditional style of marriage.

METHOD

Subjects

In order to increase varied representation of students, the participants in this study were recruited from sections of introductory religion courses that are required of all undergraduate students. Participants in this study were 100 college students (49 males, 51 females). All of the participants were single. The participants ranged in age from 17 to 33 years old (mean = 19.2, s.d. = 2.4 years).

Most (73%) were first-year students. The majority (78%) of the participants received catholic religious training, leaving 10% from protestant, 7% from other religious backgrounds, and 5% no training. They spent their childhood in suburban areas (38%), large cities (32%), from small cities (20%), from small towns (8%), and from rural communities (2%).

The subjects were placed into one of four categories according to gender and parental marital status: males with married parents (n = 38), males with divorced parents (n = 11), females with married parents (n = 38), and females with divorced parents (n = 13).

Instrument

The Marriage Role Expectation Inventory (Dunn and Debonis, 1979) served as the dependent for this study. The MREI is a three page questionnaire that consists of seventy-one questions about marriage role expectations. The questions are derived from eight major areas of interest for marriage expectations: authority, homemaking, children, personality, social participation, sexual relations, education, and employment and support. The participants respond using a Likert-type scale: strongly agree, agree, undecided, disagree, or strongly disagree. The instrument is scored in such a way that the higher the numerical value, the more companionship oriented the subject expects his or her marriage to be. The lower scores indicate that the subjects expect a traditional marriage.

The "traditional" form of marriage (Dunn, 1960) is operationally defined as a family structure containing four distinct characteristics: The male provides the primary source of income for the household, the wife's responsibilities are primarily contained in the home, she has primary responsibilities for care of the children, and the husband is to make the decisions for the household. The "companionship" role is defined as sharing the financial responsibilities, sharing responsibility of housework, both husband and wife are responsible for the care of the children, and the husband and wife share in the decision making for the household.

The first Page of the MREI contains questions which ask demographic information, including gender, age, marital status, parent's marital status, years of education, type of community in which childhood was spent, and childhood religious training.

Procedure

The researcher was granted permission to enter various sections of introductory religious studies classes on the first or second class meeting of the 1991 Fall semester. The researcher briefly introduced the study and its purpose. Those who agreed to participate were given a copy of the MREI and were asked to complete the survey immediately and then return it to the researcher. They were told that this survey was to be completed anonymously. The inventory required less that 15 minutes to complete.

RESULTS

These one hundred participants are summarized in Table 1. A somewhat negatively skewed, leptokurtic distribution of MREI total scores was obtained (mean = 292.70, s.d. = 32.74). The total MREI score was found to possess high reliabilities (alpha = .95, split-half = .87, corrected split-half = .93).

When the MREI scores were examined for sex differences, large and significant differences were observed on the total score as well as in each of the eight subscales (see Table 2).

Two-way (sex $\times$ parental marital status) ANOVAs were performed on total MREI scores and MREI subscales. The ANOVA for the total MREI revealed a significant interaction between parental marital status and gender on the total MREI score, $F(1,96) = 4.33$, $p < .05$. Significant interactions were also found for the home and child subscales. Significant mean effects for sex were found for each scale (see Table 3).

Table 4 lists the means for the total MREI scores for the four

Table 1
MREI Total and Subscale Scores

Scale	Min.	Max.	Median	Mean	S.D.
Total	145	346	295.5	292.70	32.74
Authority	17	50	41.0	40.22	5.72
Homemaking	12	45	37.0	36.53	5.35
Children	26	49	41.0	40.42	3.91
Personality	20	40	33.0	32.80	4.37
Social	16	40	32.5	32.50	4.37
Sex	16	35	27.0	26.57	3.74
Education	26	50	44.0	43.75	4.85
Employment	15	45	36 0	35.95	5.32

Table 2
Sex Differences in Mean MREI Scores

Scale	Female	Male	t	p<
Total	308.47	276.29	5.62	.001
Authority	42.78	37.55	5.13	.001
Homemaking	38.78	34.18	4.74	.001
Children	41.75	39.04	3.67	.001
Personality	34.20	31.35	3.43	.001
Social	34.23	30.80	4.26	.001
Sex	27.65	25.45	3.43	.001
Education	45.78	41.63	4.72	.001
Employment	38.71	33.08	6.21	.001

Table 3

Summary of Two-Way ANOVA F-ratio

Variable	Marital Status	Gender	Interaction
Total	<1.00	32.65***	4.33**
Authority	<1.00	27.03***	3.26
Home	<1.00	24.14***	7.23**
Children	1.56	14.54***	5.86*
Personality	<1.00	11.61***	<1.00
Social	<1.00	18.17***	2.08
Sex	1.83	12.29***	1.91
Education	<1.00	22.05***	1.33
Employ	<1.00	38.18***	<1.00

* $p < .05$ **$p < .01$

Table 4

Significant Group Differences on MREI Scales

Gender	Male	Male	Female	Female
Parental Marital Status	Married	Divorced	Married	Divorced
MREI Total	280.39	262.09	306.11	315.39
Homemaking	35.11	31.00	38.32	40.15
Children	39.76	36.55	41.53	42.38

groups: males with married parents, males with divorced parents, females with married parents, and females with divorced parents. A Newman Keuls procedure revealed that these four groups were all significantly different from ear other at the 0.05 level.

Figure 1 illustrates this interaction between gender and parents marital status on the MREI total score. For the males, higher MREI scores were found in those whose parents are still married. However, for females, the higher MREI scores were found in those from divorced families.

The lowest total MREI mean score of 262.09 came from male participants with divorced parents; the mean score for male participants with married parents was 280.39.

However, the mean total MREI score for females from divorced families was 315.38 and the mean score for the females from married parents was 306.10. Female subjects from a divorced family anticipated a more companionship oriented marriage role.

FIGURE 1. The interaction between gender/parental marital status and total MREI score.

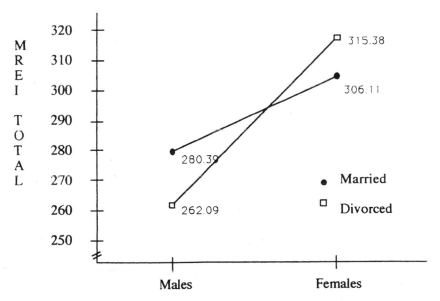

DISCUSSION

The interaction between gender and parental marital status reveals that male and female participants react differently to parental divorce. Males from divorced families reported more traditional marriage role expectations than did males from intact families. Females from divorced families reported more companionship oriented marriage role expectations than did females from intact families.

Overall gender differences ignoring the factor of parental marital status revealed that all the females in the study were more companionship oriented than all of the males. The distribution of companionship and traditional marriage role expectations clearly was not even across parental marital status groups.

What this research has added to this area is the variable of gender in the investigation of marriage role expectations and parental marital status. This is an important new variable when developing methods to study and to help children of divorce.

From the findings in this study, researchers and others working with children of divorce need to be aware of these gender differences that may be present. The present study suggests that future research of the effects of divorce needs to look for different effects in male and female children. Gender needs to be examined as a variable in the expectations that these two groups of children of divorce hold toward their own marriages.

REFERENCES

Carson, D. K., & Kelly, K. M. (1990). Perceptions of marriage and family life of young adults with and without histories of parental divorce. *Psychological Reports, 66*, 33-34.

Dunn, M. (1960). Marriage role expectations of adolescents. *Marriage and Family Living, 20*, 99-101.

Dunn, M., & DeBonis, J.N. (1979). *Teacher's and counselor's guide to the marriage role expectation inventory.* Saluda, NC: Family Life Publications.

Gabardi, L., & Rosén, L. (1991). Differences between college students from divorced and intact families. *Journal of Divorce & Remarriage, 15*, 175-191.

Ganong, L., Coleman, M., & Brown, G. (1981). Effect of family structure on marital attitudes of adolescents. *Adolescence, 16*, 281-288.

Greenberg, E., & Nay, R. (1982) The intergenerational transmission of marital instability reconsidered. *Journal of Marriage and the Family 44*, 335-347.

Kelly, J. B. (1981). Observations on adolescent relationships five years after divorce. *Adolescent Psychiatry, 9*, 133-141.

Kinnaird, K. L., & Gerrard, M. (1986). Premarital sexual behavior and attitudes toward marriage and divorce among young women as a function of their mother's marital status. *Journal of Marriage and the Family 48*, 757-765.

Long, B. H. (1987). Perceptions of parental discord and parental separations in the United States: Effects on daughters' attitudes toward marriage and courtship progress. *Journal of Social Psychology, 127*, 573-582.

Mueller, C., & Pope, H. (1977). Marital instability: A study of its transmission between generations. *Journal of Marriage and the Family, 39*, 83-93.

Southworth, S., & Schwarz, J. (1987). Post-divorce contact, relationship with father, and heterosexual trust in female college students. *American Journal of Orthopsychiatry, 57*, 371-382.

Wallerstein, J. (1987). Children of divorce: Report of a ten-year follow-up of early latency-age children. *American Journal of Orthopsychiatry, 57*, 199-211.

Weeks, M., O'Neal, & Botkin, D. (1987). A longitudinal study of the marriage role expectations of college women: 1961-1984. *Sex Roles, 17*, 49-58.

Anti-Marriage Attitudes and Motivations to Marry Amongst Adolescents with Divorced Parents

Fiona L. Tasker

SUMMARY. Results are reported from a study of white males and females aged 17-18 from different socioeconomic groups with married or divorced parents (n = 306). Teenagers from divorced backgrounds were less likely to say that they want to marry compared with teenagers from intact families. However, other indicators reveal that they may in fact marry early as they are more affected by variables associated with early marriage: leaving school; leaving home; and forming serious boyfriend/girlfriend relationships. Daughters of divorce were most affected by these pro-marriage influences. Distinctions are drawn between different groups of children of divorce and between marital attitudes and behaviour. It is suggested that the adolescent's own experience of intimate relationships and cohabitation can overcome negative attitudes to marriage arising from parental divorce.

INTRODUCTION

A number of studies have compared the attitudes to marriage of children from intact and divorced backgrounds and found that those

Fiona L. Tasker, PhD, is a Research Fellow at the Clinical and Health Psychology Research Centre, City University, Northampton Square, London. EC1V 0HB. U.K.
The study was conducted at the Child Care and Development Group, University of Cambridge, Free School Lane, Cambridge. CB2 3RF. U.K. This work was supported by an Economic and Social Research Council studentship to the author. The author would like to thank Dr. Martin Richards for his supervision of the project.

© 1992 by The Haworth Press, Inc. All rights reserved.

who have experienced their parents' divorce hold more negative views about marriage (e.g., Coleman and Ganong, 1984; Garbardi and Rosén, 1991). However, the results of these surveys have been inconsistent (Amato, 1988; Tasker and Richards, forthcoming). For example, Greenberg and Nay (1982) find that adolescents with divorced parents were not less willing to consider marriage, although they expressed more favourable attitudes to divorce.

If teenagers from divorced backgrounds do indeed have more negative views about marriage, the most obvious prediction would be that they would be less likely to marry when they enter adulthood, or at least delay marriage for longer than their contemporaries. Demographic data gives limited support to this prediction. Some adult children of divorce remain single (Kobrin and Waite, 1984). However, there is more demographic data to the contrary indicating that many children of divorce in fact marry earlier than their contemporaries from intact families (e.g., Kobrin and Waite, 1984; Kuh and Maclean, 1990; Bumpass, Sweet and Martin, 1991).

In examining the relationship between attitudes to marriage and marital behaviour it is therefore necessary to examine other factors, aside from self-reported preference for and against marriage that could lead children of divorce to an early wedding. Three factors that predict early marriage have been identified by previous studies on the timing of marriage. Leaving school at the earliest opportunity is more common amongst working class teenagers and tends to be associated with early marriage, especially for girls (Carlson, 1979; Kiernan, 1986). Leaving home is also associated with marriage. Marriage is still a major reason for leaving home, especially for working class girls (Jones, 1987). Leaving home because of unhappiness may also encourage the young person to rely on other relationships and so promote early marriage (Mansfield and Collard, 1988). Becoming involved with a steady boyfriend/girlfriend is also associated with early marriage, and girls tend to become involved in steady relationships at an earlier age than do boys (Chilman, 1983).

There is other evidence to suggest that teenagers from divorced backgrounds are more likely to be affected by these three marriage motivators. Firstly, children of divorce, and particularly the girls, are more likely to have left the education system with fewer and lower qualifications (Amato and Keith, 1991). Secondly, they tend to leave home earlier than their contemporaries (Mitchell, Wister and Burch, 1989; Kiernan, forthcoming). Finally, they are more likely to have been involved in heterosexual relationships (Flewelling and Bauman, 1990; Garbardi and Rosén, 1991), and be cohabiting (Booth, Brinkerhoff and White, 1984).

Apparently there are two opposite trends in the data on marital attitudes and behaviour of children of divorce, indicating both pro-marriage and anti-marriage inclinations. Unfortunately, neither the attitude to marriage studies, nor the demographic surveys, have concurrently measured both attitudes to marriage and whether or not the young person is in circumstances which influence the likelihood of marriage. Previous studies have not, therefore, investigated the possible reasons why these seemingly contradictory patterns occur.

Two explanations for these divergent trends in marital attitudes and behaviour merit consideration in this paper. Firstly, it is possible that some children of divorce are opposed to marriage and remain single, whilst others, presumably more pro-marriage in their attitudes than their contemporaries, marry sooner. However, it is also possible that marital attitudes and marital behaviour do not coincide so that teenagers, who have negative views about marriage, decide to marry as they enter into adulthood. Children from divorced backgrounds are, of course, likely to show a variety of attitudes and these may change rapidly over time and be a poor indicator of later behaviour. It is hypothesized that teenagers from divorced backgrounds would be more negative about marriage, but would on the other hand be more likely to find themselves in circumstances which might lead to an early marriage. It is also hypothesized that girls from divorced backgrounds, who also come from working class homes, are more likely to have left school, left home and be involved in steady relationships, since it is proposed that parental divorce is likely to accentuate the differences between the genders and socioeconomic groups where these trends are present.

METHOD

Subjects and Recruitment

Given the requirements for the study to investigate the influence of parental divorce on teenagers in the context of gender and social class, a community sample was recruited from the electoral roll in the City of Cambridge, U.K. Despite the legal requirement for all teenagers reaching their eighteenth birthday to register, Todd and Butcher (1981) estimate that approximately 24% of those eligible are not registered (mostly those from lower socioeconomic groups who are most mobile in the housing market). With the exclusion of two of the town centre electoral register wards, and one ward in which the teenagers were contacted for the purposes of a pilot study, all the attainers on the electoral roll (n = 825) in the remaining eleven electoral wards were sent a postal questionnaire in June 1988 and asked to take part in the survey. A single reminder was sent to those who did not reply to the first letter and questionnaire.

The study achieved a 40% (n = 331) response rate to the postal questionnaire. Unfortunately it was not possible to investigate the reasons for non-response. The distribution of the sample can be seen in Table 1. From this we can see that 26% of the sample had divorced parents, in comparison to Haskey's national U.K. extrapolation from demographic data that 1 in 5 teenagers are likely to have experienced parental divorce by the time they are sixteen (Haskey, 1983). Of the 85 children with divorced parents in this sample 35% currently lived with their single mother, 27% lived with their remarried mother, 14% lived with their father on his own or with his new wife, and 24% of the children with divorced parents were living away from either parent. The average age at which children reported that their parents had separated was eight and a half years (s.d. = 4.9).

Table 1 also indicates that the sample is more representative of the views of middle class teenagers and girls than it is of working class teenagers and boys. The percentages of teenagers from divorced backgrounds are distributed in approximately equal proportions between the sexes and the two social class groups. Eighteen per cent of adolescents (n = 53) reported that one or both of their parents had been born outside the U.K.

Table 1. Demographic characteristics of the total sample of Cambridge teenagers (n=331).

	Parental Marital Status			Social Class		Gender	
	Married (M.P.)	Divorced (D.P.)	Other	Middle	Working	Boys	Girls
Total	67% (221)	26% (85)	8% (25)	64% (183)	36% (103)	36% (182)	64% (104)
Divorced Parents[1]	–	–	–	24% (44)	30% (31)	26% (28)	29% (56)

[1] Ten of the children with divorced parents did not indicate their father's occupation. One of the teenagers with divorced parents did not indicate their sex on the questionnaire.

The social class measure taken was the socioeconomic group of their father. This was then coded according to the Registrar General's classification (Office of Population Censuses and Surveys, 1980), owing to small numbers, these categories were re-grouped into into non-manual and manual occupations. There is obviously some debate about the suitability of assigning social class ratings to teenagers from divorced backgrounds on the basis of their father's occupation, when in only 12/85 cases the teenagers were living with their fathers. However, a more detailed account of the household's circumstances post-divorce would have been difficult to obtain, given the decision not to involve the teenagers' parents in the study. The ten cases in which the teenagers failed to give details of their father's occupation were excluded from the analyses as missing data.

Materials

As this report only concerns the answers to a few of the questions asked in the survey, full details of the questionnaire are not presented here but can be obtained from the author (Tasker, 1990). Subjects were asked whether they wanted to marry in the future, the reasons for their choice, and whether they would consider living-together relationships. They were also asked to indicate whether they lived with either of their parents or not, whether they had left school or college, and whether they had ever had a serious or steady relationship.

Thirty-one of the teenagers were also interviewed one to three months after having returned their questionnaires. These teenagers were picked from a potential 90 interview volunteers with approximately equal numbers in each family background, social class and gender group. The teenagers' wishes to marry or remain single as expressed in these interviews were in 24/28 (86%) cases in agreement with the yes/no option checked in their questionnaires (three teenagers missed this question in the interview/questionnaire). Three teenagers were ambivalent in either the questionnaire or the interview, but were firmly in favour of marriage in the context of the other method. In only one case did the teenager change her mind from non-marriage when completing the questionnaire to pro-marriage when expressing her views in the interview. This is referred to in the discussion below.

Statistical Analysis

The variables considered in the analyses that follow are all two level categorical variables. These variables were initially analysed using Pearson's Chi-square statistic and subsequently logit models in loglinear analysis to assess possible interactions between parental marital status and gender or social class on the outcome variable.

Loglinear analysis compares the observed values to the expected values created by the proposed model of the data. The better the fit of the model to the data the smaller the resulting likelihood-ratio Chi-square statistic; the reverse of the situation in the more traditional use of Chi-square. To find out which of the terms included in the model is influencing the distribution, the individual parameter coefficients are assessed. These coefficients compare the log of each of the cell frequencies (O) with the log of the average frequencies over all cells (E). If the standardized value of the coefficient (Z) is greater than plus or minus 1.96 then statistical significance at $p < 0.05$ has been reached.

RESULTS

Attitudes to Marriage

Table 2 indicates that teenagers from divorced backgrounds are more likely to say that they do not want to marry in the future, although the majority of teenagers from divorced backgrounds obviously do still want to marry at some point. Loglinear analysis indicates that a main effects model best describes the data and that parental marital status is the only variable of the three to significantly affect whether the teenagers are pro- or anti-marriage (likelihood-ratio Chi-square = 1.525; df = 4; p = 0.822).

Why are adolescents from divorced backgrounds more negative about marriage? Survey participants were asked to list the reasons why they wanted or did not want to marry. The most common reason given for not wishing to marry was that cohabitation was a more feasible alternative 39% (14). Those who did not wish to marry were more likely to say that they would consider a cohabiting relationship (Pearson's Chi-square 3.483, df = 1, p = 0.031 one-tailed), only one person who wished to remain unmarried also said no to cohabiting. Children of divorced parents were generally more

Table 2. Influence of parental marital status, social class and gender on attitudes to marriage, leaving school and leaving home (Z scores, percentages and numbers of teenagers involved).

	Parental Marital Status		Social Class		Gender	
	Married	Divorced	Middle	Working	Boys	Girls
No to Marriage	-2.03 11% (22)	+2.03 21% (14)	+0.92 15% (25)	-0.92 12% (11)	-1.19 11% (10)	+1.19 16% (26)
Left School	-1.52 38% (80)	+1.52 51% (38)	-7.69 24% (43)	+7.69 74% (75)	+0.37 42% (43)	-0.37 41% (75)
Left Home	-4.00 6% (13)	+4.00 24% (18)	-0.42 10% (18)	+0.42 13% (13)	-2.73 4% (4)	+2.73 15% (27)

likely to say that they would consider living-together relationships, 95% versus 85% of children with married parents $z = 2.36$ (main effects model likelihood ratio chi-square $= 4.829$; df $= 4$; p $= 0.305$).

Remaining in Education

Not surprisingly the data shown in Table 2 indicate that the main demographic variable to be associated with leaving school at the minimal school leaving age is social class (loglinear analysis main effects likelihood-ratio Chi-square $= 3.352$; df $= 4$; p $= 0.501$). Teenagers whose fathers are employed in non-manual occupations are more likely to stay on at school.

The pervasive influence of social class background on children's educational attainment overshadows the reduced likelihood of teenagers from divorced backgrounds remaining at school, an association that in Table 2 remains below statistical significance. However, separate crosstabulations of the influence of parental divorce together with gender show that the girls who have experienced parental divorce are more likely to have already left school, 55% (n = 26) versus 37% (n = 49) (Pearson's chi-square $= 3.821$; df $= 1$; p $= 0.025$ one-tailed). No comparable difference is observable amongst the boys from different types of household.

Leaving Home Early

The 17-18 year olds recruited to this study were sampled prior to higher-education attendance and therefore only a small number of teenagers in the study (12%, n = 31) had left home at this stage. Of the teenagers who had left home, half (16) had also lived with their partner.

Loglinear analysis indicated that a main effects model including parental marital status, gender and social class provided the best explanation for the data (likelihood ratio Chi-square $= 3.385$; df $= 4$; p $= 0.429$). Table 2 reveals that children with divorced parents were more likely to have left home than were children from intact families. Similarly there is a main effect shown for gender, with the girls in the sample being more likely to have left home early than were the boys. The combination of both parental marital status and gender means that 33% (16) of the girls with divorced parents in the sample had left home by 17-18 in comparison with 8% (11) of the girls with married parents. No effects of social class background upon leaving home early were apparent in the data.

Boyfriends/Girlfriends: Steady Relationships

Loglinear analysis indicated that a model containing interaction effects of parental marital status and gender best explains the proportions of teenagers in each group who report having had a serious boyfriend/girlfriend relationship by age eighteen (Likelihood ratio Chi-square = 0.272; df = 1; p = 0.602). Table 3 indicates that boys are significantly less likely to report that they have been involved in

Table 3. Main effects and interaction terms showing the associations between parental marital status (P.M.S.), gender and social class and whether the teenager has had a steady relationship.

	Main Effects		Interaction Terms		
	Z score	Percent	P.M.S.	Z score	Percent
Married Parents (M.P.)	-1.39	60% (126)	-	-	-
Divorced Parents (D.P.)	+1.39	68% (55)	-	-	-
Middle Class	+0.66	66% (115)	M.P.	-1.11	59% (81)
			D.P.	+1.11	73% (41)
Working Class	-0.66	62% (66)	M.P.	-1.11	62% (45)
			D.P.	+1.11	63% (21)
Males	-2.59	56% (51)	M.P.	+2.78	61% (47)
			D.P.	-2.78	51% (14)
Females	+2.59	72% (120)	M.P.	-2.78	60% (79)
			D.P.	+2.78	85% (41)

a steady relationship than are girls. This effect is exaggerated when parental marital status is also taken into account: Girls from divorced backgrounds being those most likely to have been involved in a steady relationship, whilst boys from divorced backgrounds are least likely to declare that they have had a serious relationship.

Attitudes to Marriage and Current Behaviour

Is there any correspondence between attitudes to marriage and being in circumstances which promote early marriage? Unfortunately, small cell sizes prevent the specific consideration of anti-marriage attitudes amongst teenagers from divorced backgrounds. However, it is possible to examine the relationship between saying no to marriage and the behavioural variables associated with early marriage over the whole sample (see Table 4). If attitudes to marriage are to be supported by current behaviour, we would expect those who say they do not wish to marry to be more likely to remain in education, reside with one or both of their parents and not to have been involved in a steady relationship. This is not the case. Furthermore, adolescents who have already left home are significantly more likely to oppose marriage. There are, therefore, indications that negative attitudes to marriage do not coincide with current behaviour associated with delaying marriage or remaining single. This suggests that adolescents from divorced backgrounds are more

Table 4. Association of anti-marriage attitudes with leaving education leaving home and being involved in a steady relationship.

	Education Left School		Home Left Home		No steady Relationship	Steady Relationship
No to Marriage	13% (19)	16% (17)	12% (28)	29% (8)	16% (15)	13% (21)
		ns	p<0.05			ns

likely to be in circumstances which promote marriage, although they may hold a more negative view of marriage.

DISCUSSION

The results above indicate support for the hypothesis that teenagers from divorced backgrounds are more likely to say that they do not want to marry in the future, in comparison to teenagers whose parents' marriage has continued. In contrast to this, there is evidence which suggests that teenagers from divorced backgrounds are in circumstances in which marriage is more likely: having left school, left home and having been involved in a steady boyfriend/ girlfriend relationship.

In the introductory section two possible explanations were suggested for both anti-marriage and pro-marriage attitudes and behaviour amongst adolescents from divorced backgrounds. Firstly, that some teenagers from divorced backgrounds could be in circumstances that make an early marriage more likely, whilst others may hold anti-marriage attitudes. Secondly, that the *same* teenagers may be opposed to marriage and yet be in circumstances that promote marriage.

In support of the first explanation, it is the girls from divorced backgrounds who are often in circumstances associated with early marriage, since they are more likely to have left home early and be involved in steady relationships. Working class girls from divorced backgrounds may also be more likely to marry early, because of leaving school at the minimum leaving age, given the social class difference in remaining in education post-sixteen. However, no particular groups of children of divorce were especially likely to hold anti-marriage views. Unfortunately, a relatively small sample size means that it has not been possible to fully assess three way interactions between parental marital status, gender and social class.

It may also be the case that differences in the divorce experience are associated with varying attitudes to marriage and motivations to marry. Among other factors, parental remarriage, post-divorce conflict, parent-child relationships and the financial circumstances of the home are likely variables to influence the teenagers' views and circumstances. It is also plausible to suggest that the teenagers' views about marriage are affected by the reasons they believe explain the breakdown of their parents' marriage. For example, attributing parental divorce to incompatibility may encourage the teenager to wish to marry if the right partner can be found. These may be fruitful lines for further inquiry (Tasker and Richards, forthcoming).

There is also evidence to support the second explanation that attitudes to marriage do not coincide with current behaviour that may lead to early marriage. Holding anti-marriage views is associated with having left home, whilst those who had left school or who were involved in steady relationships do not differ in their views about marriage when compared with their peers. Longitudinal work is necessary to see whether anti-marriage attitudes are likely to change, and whether changes in the teenagers' circumstances as regards to leaving school, leaving home and becoming involved with a partner are associated with these changes.

Cohabiting may be a factor that links leaving home and having a steady relationship with marriage. Half of those who had left home had also cohabited. Furthermore, adolescents who held anti-marriage attitudes were not rejecting living-together relationships. Possibly cohabitation, which is initially envisaged as an alternative to marriage, becomes instead a prelude to marriage.

The interview data also points to the importance of personal experience of relationships and cohabiting as factors which can override the adolescent's negative impressions of marriage as formed from observation of their parents' divorce. Of the fourteen people from divorced backgrounds who were interviewed, five people had held anti-marriage views. One person held firm views opposing marriage, however, two teenagers would consider marriage if a future partner was strongly in favour and two others now wished to marry having changed their opinions after meeting their present boyfriend/girlfriend. For example, the girl quoted below comes from a working class divorced background and is now considering marriage–despite her parents' divorce.

Interviewer: Have you thought much about getting married in the future?

Interviewee: No I hadn't. Not until a couple of months ago. I
                 never thought about it at all because my mum and
                 dad had got divorced. But then my boyfriend and
                 me started talking about getting engaged and then I
                 thought, well, maybe it won't be so bad.
Interviewer: So your parents getting divorced put you off?
Interviewee: Mm, that put me off for life, it really did. I didn't
                 want to know at all. I'd seen my parents, and a lot of
                 my friends' parents, arguing. I thought I'm not get-
                 ting married and that's the end of it, and then my
                 boyfriend started softening me up a bit.

Seven other teenagers with divorced parents reported that seeing their parents separate had made them more wary about marriage, but that they wanted to marry. In half of these cases they felt that living together with a prospect husband or wife would help to ensure that a subsequent marriage would be a success. Only 2/14 teenagers with divorced parents said that their parents' relationship had no influence on their views and that they definitely wanted to marry. It is possible to suggest that the teenagers discount the negative image of marriage formed from their parents divorce and reconsider the question of marriage to a particular partner, perhaps after having initially cohabited in a trial marriage.

The greater vulnerability of children of divorce to marital difficulties and divorce has been well substantiated in the literature (e.g., Amato and Keith, 1991). Bumpass, Martin and Sweet (1991) find that the effects of parental divorce on children's marital history are mediated primarily through their earlier age at marriage and the increased likelihood of cohabitation prior to marriage. The current study suggests a pathway through adolescence from parental divorce to leaving school, leaving home and early involvement in a steady relationship, all factors that have been shown to lead to early marriage. It is also plausible to suggest that the adolescent's initially negative attitude to marriage—at variance with their subsequent marriage—may contribute to them deciding to end the marriage, if it encounters difficulties.

In conclusion the study finds that adolescents from divorced backgrounds are more likely to say that they do not wish to marry in the future. However, teenagers from divorced backgrounds, in particular the young women, were more likely to be in circumstances which are associated with early marriage, having left school at sixteen, left home early and be involved in a serious relationship. The study indicates that these three circumstances that promote marriage may overcome the adolescent's negative attitude to marriage, and that their own experience of intimate relationships, and the possibility of cohabiting with their partner, play a key role in this process. Future longitudinal work is called for to explore these interconnections.

REFERENCES

Amato, P. R. (1988). Parental divorce and attitudes toward marriage and family life. *Journal of Marriage and the Family* 50, 453-461.

Amato, P. R. and Keith, B. (1991). Parental divorce and adult well-being: A meta-analysis. *Journal of Marriage and the Family* 53, 43-58.

Booth, A., Brinkerhoff, D. B., and White, L. K. (1984). The impact of parental divorce on courtship. *Journal of Marriage and the Family* 46, 85-94.

Bumpass, L. L., Martin, T.C., and Sweet, J. A. (1991). The impact of family background and early marital factors on marital disruption. *Journal of Family Issues* 12, 22-42.

Carlson, E. (1979). Family background, school and early marriage. *Journal of Marriage and the Family* 41, 341-353.

Coleman, M. and Ganong, L. (1984). Effect of family structure on family attitudes and expectations. *Family Relations* 33, 425-432.

Chilman, C. S. (1983). Adolescent marriage and childbearing within marriage. Pp. 167-179 In *Adolescent Sexuality in a Changing American Society,* Chilman, C. S. (Ed.), Chichester: John Wiley and Sons Inc.

Flewelling, R. L. and Bauman, K. E. (1990). Family structure as a predictor of initial substance use and sexual intercourse in early adolescence. *Journal of Marriage and the Family* 52, 171-181.

Gabardi, L. and Rosén, L. A. (1991). Differences between college students from divorced and intact families. *Journal of Divorce & Remarriage* 15, 175-191.

Greenberg, E. F. and Nay, W.R. (1982). The intergenerational transmission of marital instability reconsidered. *Journal of Marriage and the Family* 44, 335-347.

Haskey, J. (1983). Children of divorcing couples. *Population Trends* 31, 20-26.

Jones, G. (1987). Leaving the parental home: An analysis of early housing careers. *Journal of Social Policy* 16, 49-74.

Kiernan, K. E. (1986). Teenage marriage and marital breakdown: A longitudinal study. *Population Studies* 40, 35-54.

Kiernan, K. E. (1991). Transitions in Young Adulthood: Effects of Family Disruption. Forthcoming, Family Policy Studies Centre, London.

Kobrin, F. E. and Waite, L. J. (1984). Effects of childhood family structure on the transition to marriage. *Journal of Marriage and the Family* 46, 807-816.

Kuh, D. and Maclean, M. (1990). Women's childhood experience of parental separation and their subsequent health and socioeconomic status in adulthood. *Journal of Biosocial Science* 22, 1-15.

Mansfield, P. and Collard, J. (1988). *The Beginning of the Rest of Your Life? A Portrait of Newly-Wed Marriage.* London: The MacMillan Press Ltd.

Mitchell, B. A., Wister, A. V., and Burch, T. K. (1989). The family environment and leaving the parental home. *Journal of Marriage and the Family* 51, 605-613.

Office of Population Censuses and Surveys. (1980). *Classification of Occupations.* London: HMSO.

Tasker, F. L. (1990). *Adolescents' attitudes to marriage and relationships following parental divorce.* Unpublished Ph.D. thesis, University of Cambridge.

Tasker, F. L. and Richards, M. P. M. (1992). The attitudes to marriage and the marital prospects of children of divorce: A review. Forthcoming, Clinical and Health Psychology Research Centre, City University, London.

Todd, J. and Butcher, B. (1981). *Electoral Registration in 1981.* London: O.P.C.S. Social Survey.

Relationships Between Divorce and College Students' Development of Identity and Intimacy

Eileen Nelson
Jamie Allison
Donna Sundre

SUMMARY. This study investigated how parental divorce during Erikson's identity stage may alter a child's ability to successfully resolve the identity and intimacy crises. Successful progression through the identity and intimacy crises was determined by the Personal Orientation Inventory (Shostrom, 1974). Family functionality during adolescence was also assessed, using the Family Adaptability and Cohesion Evaluation Scale (Olson, 1985). Subjects from homes where parental divorce occurred between the ages of 11 and 17 were compared to subjects from homes where parental divorce occurred prior to age 11 and to subjects from intact homes. The results did not yield significant differences between the groups.

Much research has been done on the topic of divorce, especially in the past twenty years. The divorce rate, steadily on the rise throughout the 1980s, has finally reached the disheartening statistic that one of every two marriages in the United States will fail (Brehm & Kassin, 1990). The National Institutes of Mental Health have stated that marital disruption is a strong predictor of physical and emotional illness (Brehm & Kassin, 1990). Divorce is not a

Eileen Nelson, EdD, is Professor of Psychology at the James Madison University, Harrisonburg, VA, 22801.

Jamie Allison is a graduate student at the James Madison University.

Donna Sundre, PhD, is Assistant Professor and Associate Assessment Specialist at the James Madison University.

© 1992 by The Haworth Press, Inc. All rights reserved.

121

single event that occurs and passes within a few weeks time. It is a process with several stages, and the effects on those involved often require much time to resolve.

The individuality of divorce situations results in difficulty generalizing the effects on children. Hetherington (1982) and Sorosky (1977) identified several factors that affect how family members react and recover from a divorce. These include the nature of the divorce, post divorce parent child relationships, age and sex of the child, the child's outside support systems and coping strategies, and other external events. Some research has found longterm, detrimental effects of divorce (DiNicola, 1989; Mueller & Pope, 1977; Wallerstein & Blakeslee, 1989). Others have found only shorterm negative effects (Hetheringinton, 1979, 1982; Parish & Wigle, 1985) and some research has found no effects or positive effects of divorce (Duberman, 1975; Kurdek & Siesky as cited in Wiehe, 1984; Lussen, 1988).

A divorce and the resulting upheaval in family structure occurs during some point in a child's psychological development. According to Erikson (1959), children experience successive developmental crises, which are separated by periods of relative equalibrium. One's personality comes about in epigentic stages, each taking place in a predetermined sequence. Significant changes, such as divorce, can be detrimental to a child's progression through these stages. Although research on the effects of divorce on children is abundant, very little attention has been paid to the impact of divorce in relation to specific developmental stages and the psychological tasks involved in those stages. This study will examine how divorce affects children's progression through Erikson's identity and intimacy crises.

IDENTITY

Identity includes a sense of self and feelings of value, adequacy and dignity as a person. According to Erikson's theory of development (as cited in Jensen, 1985), the formation of identity begins at age twelve, but is not completed until young adulthood (around age twenty-one). The psychological task at this time is to integrate the past, present and plans for the future into a whole sense of self (Elkind, 1973). During the time that identity formation is taking place, one is in psychological moratorium, which is an experimentation period (Steinberg, 1985). At this time, it is important to strongly identify with peer groups and role models because imitation of others aides the consolidation of one's own identity. It is for this reason that much of the success with identity formation is determined by a child's relationship with parents (Elkind, 1973).

INTIMACY

In addition to identity, the formation of a capacity for intimacy is another important psychological task of the young adult. Erikson called this stage intimacy versus isolation and it occurs after the identity stage is complete (Fuhrmann, 1990; Steinberg, 1985). Because intimacy involves the ability to be empathetic and to give oneself to another, it is first necessary that a strong sense of self exist. Wallerstein and Blakeslee (1989) found that children of divorce often feel rejected and abandoned by their parents. Research by Evans (1987) indicated that children who are neglected sometimes have a fear of intimacy that is countered by a fear of abandonment. They learn not to be emotionally dependent on others because their needs will not be met; however, when a relationship emerges, they will often cling to it even if it becomes abusive, rather than be alone again. Kelly (1981) found that, 5 years after a divorce, subjects who were otherwise well adjusted had not yet succeeded in maintaining healthy heterosexual relationships. Research by Lussen (1988) found the same vulnerability in intimate relationships, but she also found increased maturity, a more internal locus of control, and stronger self reliance in her subjects.

The problems associated with children of divorce are not only due to the divorce itself. Research has consistently shown that conflict and disharmony associated with the divorce process are the most upsetting aspects of divorce (McLoughlin & Whitfield, 1984; Mechanic & Hansell, 1989; Oppawsky, 1988; Slater & Haber, 1984; and Sorosky, 1977). When comparing intact versus divorced families by conflict level, Slater and Haber (1984) found that divorced families with low conflict were rated more desirable than intact families with high conflict. The high conflict homes, whether they were divorced or intact, produced more anxiety, lower self esteem, and more depression in children than did low conflict divorced and intact homes. One study by McLoughlin and Whitfield (1984) also indicated that adolescents from high conflict pre-divorce families viewed the divorce as being a "good thing," a "relief," more often than adolescents from low conflict pre-divorce homes.

High conflict is only one example of the negative impact of divorce. Research studies have examined several aspects of divorce that can initiate dysfunctional family patterns. The goal of a family is to meet the needs of it's members. When the family system is no longer accomplishing that goal, it can be termed dysfunctional (Brown & Samis, 1986). Criteria used to evaluate family functioning vary with each research study. Olson, Russell, & Sprenkle's (1984) and Olson's (1985, 1986) circumplex model of family systems was chosen for this study because it condensed many of the various concepts into three general constructs: cohesion, adaptability, and communication.

Cohesion describes the emotional bonding between family members. One aspect of this construct is the development of boundaries. Boundaries contribute to a sense of family identity by allowing members to differentiate from one another (Roberts & Price, 1985). Boundaries must be clear yet permeable. Rigid boundaries make communication difficult, thus cutting down on family support. In this case, family members disengage from the family nucleus to seek emotional nurturing elsewhere. Extremely diffuse boundaries make individual family roles ambiguous, enmeshing the family members together and preventing them from developing their own autonomy (Brown & Samis, 1986; Oppawsky, 1988). According to Evans (1987), there are a number of dysfunctional family patterns called boundary violations. They include emotional issues such as neglect or overindulgence, and other issues such as role reversal or parentification of the child.

Adaptability is the capacity of the family structure to change to accommodate the needs of it's members. Both enmeshed and disengaged families resist change, even in a positive direction (Brown &

Samis, 1986). An important part of adaptability is the interactional pattern between family members. According to Brown and Samis (1986), there are three major subsystems of this: parental, spousal, and sibling subsystems. Parental subsystems allow parents to make family decisions without outside interference. Spousal subsystems allow parents to enjoy being a couple, without parental responsibilities. Sibling subsystems allow children to resolve certain issues without parental interference. There are many types of dysfunctional interactions, including overinvolvment of the stepparent in the children's lives, and a lack of flexibility in the roles taken on by each member of the family.

Communication is a facilitating dimension between cohesion and adaptability. Functional communication is positive in nature and includes support and empathy between family members. Negative communication is dysfunctional. This may include criticism, unwillingness of family members to listen to one another and putting the child in a double bind. Double bind refers to the variety of ways children can be placed in uncomfortable situations such as parents using the child as a communication bridge, or forcing the child to reject one parent in order to be accepted by the other (Oppawsky, 1988).

There are generally two types of families that form after a divorce; the single parent family and the stepfamily. Both have potential to become dysfunctional because of their very nature. In the single parent family, the economic and emotional burdens stemming from the divorce may leave less time for parenting; less time for affection, for support, and for discipline. In short, the loss of one parent means one less adult resource on which the children can rely. Any external or internal change in a family affects all parts of the system; when one parent's role is missing, other family members must pick up the burden. A single parent can adjust to the missing parental role in several ways. Research (Nester, 1980) has shown that there is a difference between maternal and paternal roles. The father plays the instrumental role, governing the family's external goals and adaptive needs. The mother's expressive role keeps a balance between the relationships of family members to one another. The single parent could intensify his or her own role or switch roles, either way neglecting part of what the child may need. The parent may try to take on both parental roles, but this could threaten the independence of the child. For example, the child is looking to the parent for both external and internal support, the bond might become strong enough to prevent differentiation. The final alternative for the parent is to give the child a role or, in essence, to parentify the child.

The second type of post-divorce family is the stepfamily. Research comparing stepfamilies to nuclear families provides conflicting information. Many studies have found no differences between stepfamilies and first marriage families in terms of quality of family relationships or family functioning (Duberman, 1975; Bood, Wilson et al., as cited in Pink & Wampler, 1985). Research by Heatherington (1982) found that stepfamilies undergo a period of adjustment, but usually stabilize within 6 years after a divorce. Some research has found that stepfamilies are more disadvantaged than first marriage families for two reasons (Pink & Wampler, 1985; Roberts & Price, 1985). First, the role of the stepparent as a friend, an authority figure, or a parent to the child is one that is poorly defined. This becomes even more complicated if the biological parent is still in contact with the children because the two adults must somehow share these roles. Second, there is often unresolved conflict and grief from the dissolution of the original family. The main problem is that the stepparent arrives in the middle of the family's lifetime. A stepparent-child relationship is not an automatic one, as it is when parents raise a child from birth. The older children are when the stepparent enters the household, the less accepting they generally are of the step parent (Wallerstein and Blakeslee, 1989). According to Wallerstein and Blakeslee (1989) a new marriage does not usually alleviate any grief the children are feeling over the loss of their original family. The newlywed couples' need for privacy can make the children feel left out and unwanted. One half of children in remarried families do not feel welcome in their homes. There may also be jealousy on the part of the children and the stepparent as to how much time each spends with the custodial parent. In a study by Pink and Wampler (1985) on remarried and intact families with adolescents, these researchers found lower cohesion, less adaptability, less inter-member regard, and less unconditionality in the remarried families.

This study focused on how divorce during the identity stage may alter the child's ability to successfully resolve the identity crisis, as well as the intimacy crisis which follows. The instrument used to assess this was the Personal Orientation Inventory (Shostrom, 1974). The POI was chosen because it contains several subscales that directly relate to the identity and intimacy crises. As previous research has shown that family dysfunction may be more detrimental than a divorce itself, the level of functionality within a family during a specific developmental stage must be determined to assess how that also affects the formation of identity and intimacy. The level of family functionality was determined by the Family Adaptation and Cohesion Evaluation Scale (Olson, 1985). Family functionality was one independent variable with three possible levels: balanced or functional; midrange; and extreme or dysfunctional. The other independent variable was the family status of the subject. This also had three levels: intact families; families experiencing parental divorce when the subject was between the ages of 11 and 17; and families experiencing parental divorce when the subject was younger than 11 years of age. The dependent variable was the subject's score on the two main scales and various subscales of the POI. Two hypotheses were formulated: (1) There would be a main effect for the family status variable. Subjects who experienced a divorce between the ages of 11 and 17 would have lower scores on the support ratio and time ratio scales as well as the capacity for intimate contact, self regard, self acceptance, nature of man and spontaneity sub-scales of the POI than subjects from intact families or families where the divorce occurred before the subject was 11 years of age. (2) There would be a main effect for the family functionality variable. Subjects from dysfunctional families would have lower scores on the support ratio and time ratio scales as well as the capacity for intimate contact, self regard, self acceptance, nature of man and spontaneity sub-scales of the POI than subjects from functional or midrange homes. Further, the interaction would be tested to identify differential scores on the support ratio and time ratio scales as well as the capacity for intimate contact, self regard, nature of man, and spontaneity sub-scales of the POI as a result of the two independent variables.

METHOD

Participants

One hundred and thirty six student volunteers at a mid-sized Southeastern university participated in the study. By requesting family status information as part of the demographic data, participants were distributed as evenly as possible across the three groupings of the family status variable. The first group were from intact families. The two divorced groups were comprised of students who experienced divorce between the ages of 11 and 17, and students who experienced divorce before the age of 11. All the participants from the divorced groups experienced divorce before the onset of college. This was to exclude those students who may have been involved in a current divorce at the time they were surveyed. All the participants were sophomores or juniors. Freshmen were excluded to prevent a confound related to adjustment to college; while seniors were not sampled to eliminate a potential confound surrounding preparation for graduation and life after college.

Description of the Instruments

The Personal Orientation Inventory (Shostrom, 1974) is composed of 150 two-choice questions that are scored first according to the two main scales: support ratio, which measures whether a person reacts primarily to self or to others; and time ratio which measures the degree to which one lives in the present. Both of these main scales are presented as proportions; outer over inner supported, and time incompetent over time competent. The possible range of scores for the support ratio scale is 0-138 over 0-127, and for the time ratio scale 0-23 over 0-23. The questions are also scored according to the following 10 sub-scales: Self-actualizing value, existentiality, feeling reactivity, spontaneity, self regard, self acceptance, nature of man, synergy, acceptance of aggression, and capacity for intimate contact.

In addition to the two main scales, time ratio and support ratio, five sub-scales were of interest in this study because they directly related to the psychological tasks in Erikson's identity and intimacy stages. The spontaneity sub-scale related to the acceptance of one's identity and a willingness to act according to it. The self-acceptance and self-regard sub-scales also related to self certainty, as well as role experimentation. The adolescent is aware of personal strengths and weaknesses and is willing to face them as one's identity evolves. The nature of man sub-scale related to the sex polarization task in the acceptance of gender roles. The capacity for intimate contact sub-scale measured the development of intimacy which comes after the identity crisis. The POI measures a "patient's state of positive mental health" (Shostrom & Knapp, 1966, p. 193). The higher one's state of positive mental health, the more self actualized one is. A self actualized person makes full use of abilities, lives in the present frame of mind, functions autonomously and has a benevolent outlook on human nature (Fox, Knapp, & Michael, 1968).

Because the bounty of research indicated that dysfunctional patterns, not only the divorce itself may be connected with various psychological problems, the Family Adaption and Cohesion Evaluation Survey (FACES) was used to assess the level of family dysfunctionality. The FACES is based on Olson, Russell & Sprenkle's (1984) and Olson's (1985, 1986) circumplex model of family systems. There are three aspects of the family system: cohesion, adaptability and communication; but only the first two are directly assessed. The test consists of 20 questions; 10 regarding cohesion and 10 regarding adaptability. Both cohesion and adaptability are divided into four levels. These levels were determined by norms previously researched by Olson (1985). The levels for family cohesion are: disengaged, separated, connected, and enmeshed; with the two functional or balanced levels being separated and connected. The levels for family adaptability are: rigid, structured, flexible, and chaotic; with the two functional or balanced levels being structured and flexible. Putting these combinations together yields sixteen possible family systems. These combinations provided the three groups used as an independent variable in this study: functional, that is balanced on both the cohesion and adaptability dimensions; midrange, which is balanced on only one dimension; and dysfunctional, or extreme on both dimensions. Olson (1985), hypothesized that balanced families are more functional than extreme ones. Research by Olson (1985) using families with alcoholics, sex offenders, and fathers absent has supported this hypothesis.

Procedure

Participants were assigned to a family status variable based on whether their parents were divorced or married. Participants signed an informed consent form that stated they had the right to withdraw from the study at any time. Participants were assured of confidentiality through the use of number codes. The POI was taken in a present frame of reference, however, subjects were asked to take the FACES as relating to when they were between 11 and 17 years of age. This was done so that family functioning could be assessed in the time frame of the identity and intimacy crises.

Data Analysis

Subsequent to data collection each subject fit into one of nine categories based on the two independent variables: family status and family functionality. A 3 × 3 MANOVA was used to assess main effects and interactions of the independent variables. In the event that the number of subjects in the dysfunctional group was too limited, a 2 × 3 MANOVA was planned in which the dysfunctional and midrange groups would be collapsed together. In the event that the number of subjects in one or both of the divorced groups was too limited, a 2 × 3 MANOVA was planned in which the 2 divorced groups would be collapsed together.

RESULTS

One hundred and thirty six participants completed the POI and FACES inventories. Based on decisions made as described in the methods section, the participants were placed in 9 cells. Table 1 shows the distribution of subjects throughout the cells.

The main effect for the family status variable was found to be nonsignificant for all the scales [capacity for intimate contact $F(2,$

Table 1

Distribution of Subjects in Independent Variable Cells

	Family Functionality			
Family Status	Funct.	Midrange	Dysfunct.	Total
Intact	29	6	2	37
Divorce <11	37	12	6	55
Divorce 11-17	35	8	1	44
Total	101	26	9	136

Note. Funct. = Functional; Dysfunct. = Dysfunctional

127) = 1.05, $p > .05$; self regard $F(2, 127) = 2.02$, $p > .05$; self acceptance $F(2, 127) = .272$, $p > .05$; nature of man $F(2, 127) = .555$, $p > .05$; spontaneity $F(2, 127) = 1.80$, $p > .05$; time ratio $F(2, 127) = .478$, $p. > .05$; support ratio $F(2, 127) = .751$, $p > .05$].

The main effect for the family functionality variable was found to be nonsignificant for all the scales [capacity for intimate contact $F(2, 127) = .463$, $p > .05$; self regard $F(2, 127) = .645$, $p > .05$; self acceptance $F(2, 127) = .1.32$, $p > .05$; nature of man $F(2, 127) = .178$, $p > .05$; spontaneity $F(2, 127) = .264$, $p > .05$; time ratio $F(2, 127) = .943$, $p > .05$; support ratio $F(2, 127) = .030$, $p > .05$].

The interaction between the family status and family functionality variables was not found to be significant for any of the scales [capacity for intimate contact $F(4, 127) = .764$, $p > .05$; self regard $F(4, 127) = .840$, $p > .05$; self acceptance $F(4, 127) = .949$, $p > .05$; nature of man $F(4, 127) - 1.46$, $p > .05$; spontaneity $F(4, 127) = .247$, $p > .05$; time ratio $F(4, 127) = .369$, $p > .05$; support ratio $F(4, 127) = .420$, $p > .05$].

DISCUSSION

The results suggest that neither family status nor family functionality have a significant impact on the measures of personality used in this study. These findings are of interest, and may help explain the lack of evidence in the literature on the effects of divorce on adolescents engaged in identity and intimacy crises. Similar findings may have been discovered by other researchers and not submitted for publication due to nonsignificant results. As Sorosky (1977) and Hetherington (1982) noted, it is difficult to generalize the effects of divorce on children because of the multitude of factors involved. These findings, which show no detrimental effects of divorce on family dysfunctionality are contrary to some of the previously discussed research (Mueller & Pope, 1977; Pink & Wampler, 1985; Slater & Haber, 1984; Wallerstein & Blakeslee, 1989).

There are several reasons why the findings of this study may have differed from the above research. One possible reason for the lack of differences between the intact and divorced groups is that the negative effects of divorce may fade over time. Research on the longterm effects of divorce have had mixed results. Hetherington (1979, 1982) found that the major disturbing effects of divorce disappeared in female adolescents by about two years after the divorce and that most stepfamilies were able to stabilize 2 to 6 years after a divorce. The results of a study of 294 college students by Grossman, Shea and Adams (1980) indicated that participants from divorced families demonstrated significantly higher levels of ego-identity than students from intact families. Similarly, St. Clair and Day (1979) found that among senior high school females, higher identity achievement was evident in females from broken homes (disrupted by either divorce or death of one parent) as compared to females from two parent homes.

Although Wallerstein and Blakeslee (1989) found psychological problems in their subjects as long as ten years after the divorce, it should be noted that they were observing a clinical population. Given the divorce was at least 2 years past for all the current participants and that they have lived away from home for at least 1 year, it may be that the divorce and family functioning do not affect them at the present time. External events, the acquisition of support systems outside the home, and the developing maturity of the participants must also be considered as factors in their adjustment (Hetherington, 1982; Sorosky, 1977).

There were several limitations in this study. One such limitation was the small number of subjects, especially from the divorced groups. The FACES instrument was not used in the method preferred by it's authors. It was designed to be completed by each member of the family in order to get a more accurate and unbiased account of family functioning. The FACES is also usually taken in the present frame of reference; however, since the time period of interest in this study was the ages of eleven and seventeen, all subjects were asked to answer the questions in reference to that time period.

In future studies of this sort, it may be helpful to use a test which focuses on one or two specific constructs rather than breaking down a general test of self actualization such as the POI. Also, additional demographic data about the current family situation may have provided important information. Details about whether their parents ever remarried or how happy the participants were in their homes at the present time were not considered in this study.

The results of this study have added to the body of research on the effects of divorce which are both extremely diverse, and often conflicting. If the divorce rate remains constant, research in this area will continue to be vital to mental health professionals, so that they may better understand how it affects those involved. These results have positive implications about children's ability to overcome family dysfunctionality and divorce to become normally functioning and productive young adults.

REFERENCES

Brehm, S., & Kassin, S. M. (1990). *Social psychology.* Boston, Mass: Houghton Mifflin Co.

Brown, N. D., & Samis, M. (1986). The application of structural family therapy in developing the binuclear family. *Mediation Quarterly, 14/15,* 86-87.

DiNicola, V. F. (1989). The child's predicament in families with a mood disorder. *Psychiatric Clinics of North America, 12,* 933-949.

Duberman, L. (1975). *The reconstituted family: A study of remarried couples and their children*. Chicago: Nelson Hall.

Elkind, D. (1973). Erik Erikson's eight ages of man. In *Annual editions, readings in psychology*. Guilford, CT: Dushkin Publishing.

Erikson, E., H. (1959). Growth and crises of the healthy personality. *Psychological Issues, 1*, 50-101.

Evans, S. (1987). Shame, boundaries and dissociation in chemically dependent, abusive and incestuous families. *Alcoholism Treatment Quarterly, 4*, 155.

Fox, J., Knapp, R. R., & Michael, W. B. (1968). Assessment of self actualization of psychiatric patients: Validity of the personal orientation inventory. *Educational and Psychological Measurement, 28*, 565-569.

Fuhrmann, B., S. (1990). Personality development. In B. S. Fuhrmann, *Adolescence, adolescents* (pp. 356-357). Glenview, Illinois: Scott Foresman.

Hetherington, M., E. (1979). Divorce: A child's perspective. In S. Chess & A. Thomas (Eds.), *Annual progress in child psychiatry and child development* (pp. 277-291). New York: Brunner/Mazel, Inc.

Hetherington, M., E., Cox, M., & Cox, R. (1982). Effects of divorce on parents and children. In M. E. Lamb (Ed.), *Nontraditional Families* (pp. 233-288). Hillsdale, NJ: Lawrence Erlbaum Assoc.

Jensen, L., C. (1985). The developing self. In L. C. Jenson, *Adolescence: theories, research, applications* (p. 70-75). St. Paul, Minn: West Publishing Co.

Kelly, J. (1981). Observations on adolescent relationships five years after divorce. *Adolescent Psychiatry, 9*, 133-142.

Lussen, L., B. (1988). The female adolescent's unconscious experience of parental divorce. *Smith College Studies in Social Work, 58*, 101-121.

McLoughlin, D., & Whitfield, R. (1984). Adolescence and their experience of parental divorce. *Journal of Adolescence, 7*, 155-170.

Mechanic, D., & Hansell, S. (1989). Divorce, family conflict and adolescent's well being. *Journal of Health and Social Behavior, 30*, 105-116.

Mueller, C. W., & Pope, H. (1977). Marital instability: A study of it's transmission between generations. *Journal of Marriage and the Family*, 83-92.

Nester. M. J. (1980). *Role change and dysfunctionality in single parent families*. U.S. International University, San Diego.

Olson, D. H., (1985). FACES III, family adaptability and cohesion scales. In Olson, D. H., *Family Inventories*, (pp. 1-142). unpublished manuscript.

Olson, D. H. (1986). Circumplex model VII: Validation studies and FACES III . *Family Process, 25*, 337-351.

Olson, D. H., Russell, C. S. & Sprenkle, D. H. (1984). Circumplex model of marital and family systems: VI theoretical update. *Family Process, 22*, 69-83.

Oppawsky, J. (1988). Family dysfunctional patterns during divorce-from the view of the children. *Journal of Divorce, 12*, 139-152.

Parish, T., S., & Wigle, S., W. (1985). A longitudinal study of the impact of parental divorce on adolescents' evaluations of self and parents. *Adolescence, 20*, 239-244.

Pink, J., & Wampler, K. S. (1985). Problem areas in stepfamilies: Cohesion, adaptability, and the stepfather-adolescent relationship. *Family Relations, 34,* 327-335.

Roberts, T. W., & Price, S. J. (1985). A systems analysis of the remarriage process: Implications for the clinician. *Journal of Divorce, 9,* 1-25.

Shostrom, E. L. (1974). *Manual for the personal orientation inventory.* San Diego, CA: Educational and Industrial Testing Service.

Shostrom, E. L., & Knapp, R. R. (1966). The relationship of a measure of self actualization (POI) to a measure of pathology (MMPI) and to therapeutic growth. *American Journal of Psychotherapy, 20,* 193-202.

Slater, E. J., & Haber, J. D. (1984). Adolescent adjustment following divorce as a function of familial conflict. *Journal of Consulting and Clinical Psychology, 52,* 920-921.

Sorosky, A. D. (1977). The psychological effects of divorce on adolescents. *Adolescence, 12,* 123-135.

Steinberg, L. (1985). Intimacy. In U. Bronfenbrenner (Ed), *Adolescence* (pp. 304-334). New York: Alfred A. Knopf Inc.

Wallerstein, J., & Blakeslee, S. (1989). *Second chances: Men, women, and children a decade after divorce.* New York: Ticknor & Fields.

The Long-Term Effects
of Parental Divorce
on Family Relationships and the Effects
on Adult Children's Self-Concept

James A. Holdnack

SUMMARY. Past research suggests that the quality of family relationships after parental divorce has an impact on the children's psychological adjustment to the divorce. Research examining the long-term effects of parental divorce on children's self-concept are equivocal. The present study examines the indirect effects of parental divorce on self-concept via changes in the family environment. Two hypotheses were tested: adult children from divorced homes would report less positive family environments, and family environment would be positively correlated with self-concept. A sample of 147 subjects from a large northeastern university were used to test the hypotheses. The results indicate that adults who experienced parental divorce or separation perceived their family of origin as emotionally distant and more disorganized than subjects whose parents were not divorced. The perception of family closeness was positively correlated with self-concept. These results suggest that the lack of family closeness after divorce may affect the children's long-term psychological adjustment.

James A. Holdnack, BA, is a doctoral student in the Counseling Psychology Program at the State University of New York at Buffalo.

Requests for information should be addressed to Mr. James A. Holdnack State University of New York at Buffalo, Department of Counseling and Educational Psychology, 409 Baldy Hall, Amherst, NY 14260.

A special thank you is extended to James C. Hansen, PhD, of the State University of New York at Buffalo for all of his advice and support.

© 1992 by The Haworth Press, Inc. All rights reserved.

INTRODUCTION

The psychological implications of the divorce process have been a major interest of researchers during the past thirty years. This increasing interest in studying the effects of divorce was related to the rapidly growing divorce rate in the United States and to concerns about the psychological impact that divorce may have on a growing number of children who will experience the divorce of their parents (Goetting, 1981). Past researchers have attempted to study the psychological adjustment and well-being of children of divorce.

The concept of self-esteem has been utilized as one measure of psychological adjustment. Past research has linked parental divorce with lower levels of self-esteem in children (Holman & Woodroofe, 1988; Long, 1986; Wiehe, 1984 and Wallerstein & Blakeslee, 1989). However, these results are not conclusive since other researchers have failed to find significant differences between children from intact homes and children who have experienced parental divorce (Amato, 1988; Amato & Ochiltree, 1987; Johnson, Hutchinson, 1988; Kanoy, Cunningham, White & Adams, 1984; Parish, 1981; Partridge & Kolter, 1987; Swartzberg, Shmukler & Chalmers, 1983 and Wyman, Cowen, Hightower & Pedro-Carroll, 1985). The inconsistent research results, regarding the impact of parental divorce on children's self-esteem, have made it difficult to predict the outcome of divorce for children (Emery, 1982; Goetting, 1981).

The failure of past research to converge upon consistent results suggests that differences in methodology and sampling may influence outcomes achieved. Also, the past inconsistencies suggest that divorce is a complex process in which intervening or moderator variables may exist. One example of a possible intervening variable is the nature of family relationships after the divorce. The primary question of whether the divorce process has an effect on children's self-esteem may not be answerable without examining mediating factors. Examination of available research implies the existence of such intervening factors.

The differential effects of divorce on children's self-esteem may be attributable to events which precede or are antecedent to the divorce. Divorce is often preceded and followed by parental and family conflict. Research has shown reduced levels of self-esteem in children from homes associated with higher levels of family and marital conflict (Bishop et al., 1989; Burt, Cohen & Bjork, 1988; Cooper, Holman & Braithwaite, 1983; Holman et al., 1988; and Swartzberg et al., 1983); from unhappy homes versus happy homes (Long, 1986 and Parish, 1981); and from rejecting versus accepting homes (Berg & Kelly, 1979). Other researchers have found that children's self-esteem is positively correlated with a supportive family environment (Amato, 1986; Buri, Kirchener & Walsh, 1987, Hoelter & Harper, 1987). Klein, Johnston and Tschann (1991) indicate that marital conflict affects a child's post-divorce adjustment indirectly through changes in the mother-child relationship. The quality of family interactions appears to play a significant role in the development of self-esteem in children (Amato & Olchiltree, 1986; Amato & Olchiltree, 1987; Kanoy et al., 1984; Partridge et al., 1987). Presumably, if changes occurred in the family environment as a result of parental divorce, the development of the child's sense of self will be affected.

The following post divorce factors have been associated with differential outcomes in children from divorced families. The continuation of parental conflict after the divorce has been associated with deleterious effects for the children (Emery, 1982; Goetting, 1981 and Peck, 1989). A statement derived from a synthesis of previous research reveals that the ability of parents to put differences aside and cooperate in child rearing and the establishment of quality relationships between each parent and their children will result in more positive outcomes for the children (Greene & Leslie, 1988; Kanoy et al., 1984; Peck, 1989; Stolberg and Bush, 1985 and Wallerstein and Blakeslee, 1989). Wallerstein et al. (1989) reports that the best outcome for the child is when both parents are committed to the child's well-being and development.

Most of the research on the effects of parental divorce on children has focused on children between the ages of 6 and 15. However, negative changes in family relationships may result in prolonged periods of conflict and stress which may have long term effects on the child's self-esteem. Although few longitudinal studies examining the effects of parental divorce on self-concept exist, the research that has been performed indicates that parental divorce has long-term detrimental effects. Wallerstein et al. (1989) observed that children of divorce experience poor self-concepts even fifteen years after the divorce of their parents.

Research on adult children of divorce has found no difference in self-esteem in adult children of divorce compared to adult children from intact families (Amato, 1988; Long, 1986 and Parish, 1981). Amato and Keith (1991), utilizing meta-analysis, determined that there is a small but consistent effect of parental divorce on adult well-being. However, they did not find a significant effect of parental divorce on adult self-concept. This conclusion was based on three studies (Amato et al., 1991). The results of the cross-sectional research studies have failed to consider the presence of intervening variables such as perceived family environment on the development of self-esteem in children of divorce.

The present study examines the effects of parental divorce on the self-concept of adults. The study is based on the following premises which are derived from previous research: divorce is a process which may negatively alter family relationships, and a person's self-concept is related to the family environment in which they were raised. It is hypothesized that parental divorce will effect self-concept indirectly through poorer family relationships.
The following hypotheses will be tested:

1. Adult children of divorce will perceive the relationships in their family of origin less positively than adult children from intact families.
2. Adult self-concept will be correlated with the perception of the family environment in the family of origin. A negative perception of family environment will be associated with lower levels of self-esteem. Positive perceptions of family environment will be associated with higher levels of self-esteem.

METHOD

Sample

The sample was comprised of undergraduate and graduate students at a large northeastern university. Subjects were enrolled as either full-time day students, full-time evening students or part-time evening students. Subjects were enrolled in courses in sociology, psychology, statistics, and social work. Participation in the research was voluntary, extra credit points were offered to subjects participating in the research project.

The sample was comprised of 147 subjects of whom 107 were female, 38 male and 2 did not specify. The sample was comprised of 61% of Ss reporting having married parents, 18% divorced parents, 3.5% separated, and 13.5% widowed. The average age at which Ss parents divorced was 12.5 with a range of 2 to 37 years old. The Ss ranged in age from 18 to 72 with an average age of 25. The racial composition of the sample included: 85% caucasian, 7% African American and 4% Asian. The marital status of the subjects included 63% single, 29% married and 6% divorced. The sample was comprised of 30% of the Ss reporting having children of their own and 31% reporting that they currently lived with their parents. The median current income level of the Ss family of origin was $40,000 with 6% earning above $100,000/year and 2.5% earning less than 10,000/year. Missing values account for percentages which do not sum to 100%.

MEASURES

Family Environment Scale

This scale measures general family climate and was developed by Moos and Moos (1981). The scale has been used widely by researchers in related studies. Burt, Cohen and Bjork (1988) found children's psychological adjustment was significantly correlated to scores on the family environment scale. The child's perception of family conflict and interpersonal control was related to negative psychological outcomes for the child.

There are ninety items which are used to derive ten subscales: cohesion, conflict, expressiveness, independence, achievement orientation, active recreational orientation, moral-religious emphasis, organization, control, and incongruence.

Reported reliabilities for the subscales range from alpha = .61 to

.78 and for this study reliabilities ranged from alpha = .54 to .84. Test-retest reliabilities have been reported as ranging from .68-.72 for 8 weeks and .52-.89 for 12 months.

Tennessee Self-Concept Scale

The Tennessee Self-Concept scale is comprised of a total self-esteem score, a self-criticism score, a definiteness about the self-concept score and eight subscales. The subscales are as follows: identity, self-satisfaction, behavior, physical self, moral-ethical self, personal self, family self, and social self. The internal reliability of the self-concept scales in this sample ranged from alpha = .73 to .94. Buri et al. (1987) reports high levels of test-retest reliability (.92) in previous studies. The Tennessee Self-Concept scale possesses strong psychometric properties and has been used extensively to measure self-esteem in previous research.

Procedure

Ss were presented with all of the measures in a random fashion and were asked to complete each measure as presented to them. Ss were instructed to refer to their family of origin when answering the Family Environment Scale. Ss were informed that if they did not understand a question they could ask the test administrator for clarification. The test administrator was not blind to the hypotheses. Subjects were assured that their answers were confidential and that no one would have access to the questionnaires except the experimenter. Subjects were debriefed about the nature and purpose of the study after completing the instruments.

RESULTS

Factor Analysis of the Family Environment Scale

Factor analysis was performed on the ten subscales of the family environment scale. This procedure was utilized to reduce the quantity of independent variables which increased the power and parsimony of the data analysis. The researcher was interested in the basic interaction patterns measured by the family environment scale and not the specific scale content. By utilizing factor analytic techniques, it was possible to extract three types of interaction patterns in the family of origin. All statistical analyses were performed using spss-x release 4.0.

Image factor extraction and varimax rotation yielded the best structural solution. Using a criteria of Eigenvalues > 1 and scree plot analysis, three factors were extracted. Table 1 presents the factor loadings of each of the ten subscales on the three rotated factors, the derived communalities of each of the subscales, and the internal reliability of each of the derived factors.

The first factor was comprised of those subscales which were related to positive family interactions: cohesion, expressiveness, independence, intellectual and cultural activity, and active recreational interactions. This factor was negatively correlated with conflict and control. The factor measures perceptions of positive family closeness, which is based on communication, engagement in cultural, intellectual and recreational activities without negative percep-

Table 1: Communalities and Factor Loadings of the Family
Environment Subscales and the Factor Reliabilities

Subscale	Communality	CLS-S	ORG-S	CTRL-S
Cohesive	.54	.66	.32	-.06
Expressive	.49	.69	.04	-.11
Conflict	.36	-.38	-.31	.35
Independence	.28	.46	.20	-.16
Achievement	.21	.06	.16	.43
Intell/Cult	.40	.57	.19	.18
Active/Rec	.47	.64	.19	.17
Moral/Relig	.09	.09	.28	.06
Organization	.28	.09	.51	.11
Control	.39	-.46	.19	.38
Cronbach's Alpha		.92	.85	.79

Note: Factors were derived with image extraction and
varimax rotation. Factors were chosen based on
Eigen values > 1. CLS-S=Closeness Scale,
ORG-S=Organization Scale, CTRL-S=Control Scale

tions of conflict and enmeshment. This scale will be referred to as the closeness scale (CLS-S), reflecting the positive, affective, cohesive interactions which it measures.

The second factor was comprised of subscales positively related to family organization and cohesiveness and negatively correlated with family conflict. This factor appears to be measuring a form of structural cohesive family organization rather than an affective cohesiveness. This scale measures how well the family works together to achieve its goals and will be referred to as the organization scale (ORG-S).

The third factor was comprised of negative perceptions of the subject's family as it was positively correlated with conflict, control and achievement orientation. This factor measures the perceptions of the parents as controlling, having high expectations of the children to achieve, and the presence of interpersonal conflict and tension. This factor reflects the perception that parents are overbearing which results in family conflict. This factor will be referred to as the controlling scale (CTRL-S).

The results of the factor analysis reveal that two of the subscales are related to more than one factor. The cohesiveness subscale appears to be related to two different types of cohesiveness. The first type of cohesiveness appears to be related to the emotional bonding among family members. The second type of cohesiveness reflects a form of cooperativeness and an ability of the family to work together as a unit. The conflict scale was related to all three of the factors. Conflict was negatively correlated to both closeness and organization, which suggests that interpersonal conflict that affects emotional bonds among family members is different from conflict which interferes with cooperative, family, task performance. A third form of interpersonal conflict emerged as a type of conflict which is a resistance to the perceived controlling behaviors of the parent.

These conceptual distinctions suggest that one cannot simply measure family cohesiveness or family conflict. These constructs are too global and do not capture the different forms of conflict and cohesion which may provide more information about the interaction patterns within the family.

A factor score was computed for each subject for all of the factors by regression of each subscale's factor loading on each of the factors. The factor scores were expressed as standard scores with a mean of 0 and standard deviation of 1.

Comparisons of Subjects from Married, Divorced, Separated and Widowed Families

Multivariate Analysis of Covariance was utilized to test the hypothesis that adult children whose parents are divorced versus those from non-divorced families would perceive their family of origin differently. Mean differences among parents' marital status groups were analyzed controlling for the effects of sex, age, race, subject's marital status, SES, birth order, and whether the subject has children.

The subjects whose parents were divorced exhibit lower mean scores on all three of the family factors as displayed in Table 2A. To test whether the pattern of mean differences was related to actual group differences or due to chance factors, a Multivariate Analysis of Covariance was performed. Table 2B displays the multivariate, univariate and post hoc analyses.

The results indicate that subjects whose parents are divorced perceive their family of origin as less close and less organized than subjects whose parents are married or widowed.

In order to examine the direct effects of family structure on self-esteem, mean differences between the groups were analyzed using the same procedure described for the comparison of differences in the perception of the family environment. The results of the MANCOVA indicate that there are no significant differences between subjects from married, divorced, separated, and widowed families on the total self-esteem scores, Wilk's Lamda = .93, multivarite $F (9,260.56) = .93$, $p > .05$ and on the self-concept subscales Wilk's Lamda = .63, multivariate $F (42, 486.56) = 1.25$, $P > .05$.

Correlation and Regression Analyses

Correlation and regression procedures were employed to test the hypothesis that perceptions of one's family of origin would be correlated with total self-concept. Table 3A displays the zero-order

Table 2A: Means and Standard Deviations of Family Environment
Factors by Parental Marital Status Groups

Parents Status	N	CLS-S	ORG-S	CTRL-S
Married	71	.034 (.775)	.109 (.479)	.044 (.563)
Divorced	19	-.429 (.975)	-.423 (.819)	-.083 (.557)
Separated	5	.156 (.655)	-.315 (.753)	.421 (.583)
Widow(er)	15	-.112 (.848)	.241 (.382)	.100 (.572)
Total	110	-.060 (.826)	.016 (.591)	.047 (.558)

Note: Factor Scores were produced using a regression procedure
with factor loadings. CLS-S=Closeness Scale, ORG-S=
Organization Scale, and CTRL-S=Control Scale

Table 2B: MANCOVA on Family Factors by Parents Marital Status

Effect	Wilks	Multivarite F	Sig.	Univariate F	Sig.
Parents Status	.76	3.05 (9,236)	.000	CLS-S 3.0	.034
				ORG-S 4.9	.003
				CTRL-S 1.5	.216

Bonferroni Post Hoc Analysis	Groups		Dependent	T-Value	Sig.
	Married VS. Divorced	CLS-S	2.20	.04
	Separated VS. Divorced	CLS-S	1.88	.06
	Widow(er) VS. Divorced	CLS-S	2.55	.01
	Married VS. Divorced	ORG-S	3.46	.00
	Separated VS. Divorced	ORG-S	.76	.45
	Widow(er) VS. Divorced	ORG-S	3.01	.00
	Married VS. Divorced	CTRL-S	.56	.57
	Separated VS. Divorced	CTRL-S	1.48	.14
	Widow(er) VS. Divorced	CTRL-S	1.57	.15

Note: Covariates used include sex, age, marital status, ses,
race, birth order, and if the subject has children or not.

Table 3A: Correlation Matrix of Total Self-Esteem Scores

w/family Environment Factors and Demographics

	Age	Race	SES	Par	Mar	CLS-S	ORG-S	CTRL-S	Total	Def
Age										
Race	-.18*									
SES	-.37**	-.18*								
Par	.21*	-.05	-.05							
Mar	.55**	-.09	-.31**	.10						
CLS-S	-.21*	-.11	.37**	-.12	-.20*					
ORG-S	.19*	-.21*	.16	-.13	.08	.27**				
CTRL-S	-.03	.04	.28**	-.15	.07	-.12	.17*			
Total	.27**	-.10	-.07	-.06	.24**	.31**	.18*	-.16		
Def	.11	-.01	.04	-.08	.15	.18*	.10	.00	.67**	
Crit	-.05	-.16	.12	.04	.09	-.23**	.00	.13	-.18*	.12

p<.05 * p<.01 ** N=128 to 146

Par=Parents marital status, Mar=Subjects Marital Status,

SES=Parents SES level, CLS-S=Closeness Scale,ORG-S=Organization

Scale, CTRL-S=Control Scale, Total=Total self-esteem score,

Def=definiteness of self-concept, Crit=Self-criticism scale

Pearson Product Moment Correlations between important demographic variables, family environment factors and the measures of self-concept.

Multivariate Multiple Regressions were performed to provide a protected F test which controlled for the large number of significance tests being performed on highly correlated dependent variables. The independent variables were entered hierarchically into the multivariate equation in the following order: sex; age; SES; race; parent's marital status; subject's marital status; does the subject have children; birth order; does the subject live with parents; three interaction variables, marital status by does the subject have children, race by SES, parents marital status by race, parents marital status by SES; and the three family environment factors. This order of entry controls for the sum effects of all the demographic variables and shows the unique contribution of the family factors to the total self-esteem measures. Multivariate F statistics were based upon Wilk's Lamda for all of the analyses.

The results of the multivariate analysis with the three total self-esteem scores as dependent variables yielded several significant variables: age, multivariate $F(3,92) = 3.42$, $p < .05$; race, multivariate $F(3,92) = 2.84$, $p < .05$; subject's marital status, multivariate $F(3,92) = 3.56$, $p < .05$ and family factor #1, multivariate $F(3,90) = 8.25$, $p < .01$. Note that the degrees of freedom differ for the family factors as they were entered after all the demographics had been entered in two stages; first entered was sex, then all of the other demographics were entered.

The variables that achieved multivariate significance were entered into Hierarchical Univariate Multiple Regressions. The Univariate Hierarchical Multiple Regression equations were derived by entering the variables in two steps: the demographic variables were entered first and the family factors were entered second. This procedure was performed to control for the common effects between the demographic variables and the family environment variables which results in a refined test of the effects of family environment. The results of the analyses appear in Table 3B.

The results of the univariate hierarchical regression show a strong positive correlation between family of origin closeness and the three total self-esteem scores. These results support the hypothesis that self-esteem is highly correlated with the subject's perception of the interactions within their family of origin, controlling for the effects of age, race and marital status.

DISCUSSION

The results of the between-group-analysis support the hypothesis that parental divorce influences the subject's perception of the interactions in their family of origin. Main effects were not found relating parental divorce to adult children's self-concept. These results are similar to previous studies which failed to find a main effect of family structure on children's self-concept (Amato, 1988; Amato et al., 1987; Johnson et al., 1988; Kanoy et al., 1984; Parish, 1981; Partridge et al., 1987; Swartzberg et al., 1983 & Wyman et al., 1985). However, these results differ from the findings of other studies (Holman et al., 1988; Parish et al., 1980 & Wiehe, 1984). The differences noted may be due to the variability in outcomes associated with divorce. The results of this study suggest that the

Table 3B: Hierarchical Univarite Multiple Regression Analysis with
3 Total Self-Esteem Scores as Dependent and Independent
variables which Achieved Multivariate Significance.

Step	D.V.	Predictor	R^2	R^2 Change	F Change	Beta
1	Total	Mar				.16
		Race				.03
		Age	.09**	.09	4.18**	.30**
2		CLS-S	.25**	.16	25.88**	.42**
1	D-Score	Mar				.01
		Race				.10
		Age	.03	.03	1.25	.22*
2		CLS-S	.09*	.06	8.41**	.26**
1	Self-Cr	Mar				.14
		Race				-.19*
		Age	.05	.05	2.31	-.25*
2		CLS-S	.13*	.08	10.42**	-.28**

note: Standardized Beta weights are derived from the final
equation

*P<.05. **P<.01.

psychological adjustment of children of divorce is strongly related
to family interactions in homes where the parents are divorced.

Although a main effect was not found for parental divorce on
self-concept, subjects from divorced homes viewed their families as
more emotionally distant than children from non-divorced families.
Perceived closeness in the family of origin was strongly correlated
with subject's self-concept across several domains. These domains
include a lack of certainty about self-attributes, and global perceptions of self-worth.

Subjects whose parents are divorced not only perceive their families as more emotionally distant than subjects whose parents are not
divorced, they also perceive their family of origin as being more

disorganized. Although family organization was not correlated with the subject's self-esteem, it may affect the subject's life in other domains not measured in this study. Family disorganization may affect the subject's ability to participate in activities outside of school or relationships outside the family. These activities require the family to be organized enough to be able to transport the child and the child may have less time to engage in these activities due to the increased responsibility of helping the family organize daily tasks and chores.

Stoltenberg, and Rosko (1991) report that the impact of lack of parental involvement is beneficial to the process of separation and individuation. They report higher levels of positive self-efficacy among students with divorced parents versus students of non-divorced families. However, the present study did not find a significant difference between subjects whose parents are divorced and subjects whose parents are not divorced on perceived controlling behavior. Both groups reported equal levels of coercive behaviors in the family. The increased self-efficacy in subjects whose parents are divorced may be a product of the subjects having to be more responsible for themselves. Therefore, they may be more confident and competent in performing self-care tasks but they may feel less confident about their self-worth which may interfere with their ability to establish and maintain intimate relationships.

Although the cause of the emotional and interpersonal distance reported by many of the subjects from divorced families was not studied directly, past research provides insight into the dynamics which affect parental involvement with their children. The level of the mother's adjustment after the divorce has a strong effect on the parent-child relationship (Copeland, 1985; Greene et al., 1988; and Stolberg et al., 1985). Kline et al. (1991) report that the mother's adjustment and her relationship with her children was negatively affected by the presence of continued marital conflict after the divorce. The mother-child relationship was also affected by the economic status of the family after the divorce (Kline et al., 1991). Concerns over financial matters coupled with the need for the single parent to work are likely to reduce the energy and resources the parent has to engage in activities with their child. Wallerstein et al. (1989) reports that the best long-term outcomes for children of divorce occur when both parents are committed to the well-being of the child and are able to put their differences aside to facilitate a positive relationship between the parents and the children.

The theoretical implication of this research is based on the finding that the divorce process often leads to a decrease in the emotional closeness between parent and child. Children feel distanced from their parents and may interpret this as rejection. Social modeling is one hypothesis that may explain the child's negative self-perceptions. The child does not treat him or herself in a positive fashion as a result of modeling the behavior of their parents. This suggests that children learn how to interact with themselves by observing how parents interact with themselves.

Another hypothesis suggests that the child tries to understand the parent's perceived rejection by attributing the cause of the rejection to personal qualities. The child assumes the blame for the poor relationship with the parent. The use of self-blame increases the child's perception that they are in control of this uncontrollable situation but also results in low self-esteem. A third hypothesis based on object relations theory would suggest that premature separation of the parent-child bond produces a sense of anxiety and uncertainty about the self-object and other-objects.

The results suggest that parental divorce has a long term effect on family relationships which indirectly affects self-concept of the children of divorce. Children from divorced families report less emotional closeness, less family organization, and equal amounts of controlling behaviors in their family of origin. The results indicate that although children of divorce in general report poorer family relations, there are some subjects who report that they have a cohesive relationship with their family even after a divorce has occurred. Children from families who are able to maintain cohesive parent-child relationships after parental divorce have a better chance of adjusting to the new family structure with their self-image intact than those children whose parents become uninvolved with them.

Clinically, the outcomes of this research indicate that family therapists need to focus on the closeness of the parent-child relationship. Treatment should address the effects of interpersonal distance and its effects on the adjustment of the child. The research results suggest that focusing on developing a working relationship between mother and father may benefit both the parents and the children. The working relationship of the therapist and the clients may serve as a social model for the process of such a relationship. It may be helpful for the parents to devise a contract that specifies ground rules for their interactions with each other when they need to communicate about and with their children.

Therapy should focus on establishing social and economic supports for the custodial parent. The presence of economic and social support will allow the custodial parent more freedom from stress which will enhance their ability to establish a cohesive and active relationship with the child. The therapist can help the non-custodial parent by reframing their support of the custodial parent as a means of helping the children.

It would be beneficial for therapy to address the role of the non-custodial parent. These parents need to understand that they play a vital role in the welfare of the child and that their absence from a relationship with the child has negative consequences. It may be helpful for the therapist to reframe the parents attempts to punish one another, either through the interference of the relationship between one of the parents and the child or through the lack of financial support, as punishment for their children.

There are several limitations to the present study. The sample in this study may not be representative of people in general. The small sample of males and minorities suggests that the results may generalize to a limited population until further research is performed.

A second limitation of the study is a reliance on self-report measures. Some of the relationship between the measures may be attributable to method effects. A third limitation of the study is the inability to make definitive statements about causality. It is possible that poor self-concept results in the subject perceiving family relationships as negative rather than vice versa. However, this would not explain the group differences in perception of family relationships. Future studies need to use larger samples so that structural model procedures can be adequately utilized. There is a need to establish temporality through longitudinal research to confirm a causal relationship between family relationships and self-concept.

A fourth limitation in this study is the use of factor scores to indicate family environment. The factor loadings of the subscales may not be stable. Future studies may need to establish the constancy of the Family Environments scales factor structure across samples and to create unit weighted total scores rather than factor scores.

The results of this research clearly display the importance of positive family interactions in the development of self-esteem in children. The literature reports mixed results relating the effects of parental divorce on the children's self-esteem. This study suggests parental divorce negatively influences the children's self-esteem when the divorce interrupts the emotional closeness between the children and the parents. However, the effects of parental divorce are not the same for all children. The difficulty in finding group differences in self-esteem between children from divorced homes versus intact homes is related to the problem of within group variance, which accounts for the inconsistent results found in previous research.

Clearly, not all children whose parents are divorced have low self-esteem nor do children from intact homes have unilaterally high self-esteem. However, there is a greater potential for children with divorced parents to develop low self-esteem as a result of disruptions in the interpersonal closeness within the child's family. As a group, children whose parents become divorced report fewer positive family interactions than children from non-divorced families. These results indicate the importance of cooperative post-divorce parenting which allows both parents to maintain a close and active relationship with their children.

REFERENCES

Allen, Sandra F., Stoltenberg, Cal D. & Rosko, Charlotte K. (1991). Perceived Psychological Separation of Older Adolescents and Young Adults From their Parents: A Comparison of Divorced Versus Intact Families. *Journal of Counseling and Development, 69*, 57-61.

Amato, Paul R. and Keith, Bruce. (1991). Parental Divorce and Adult Well-Being: A Meta-Analysis. *Journal of Marriage and the Family, 53*, 43-58.

Amato, Paul R. (1988). Long-term implications of parental divorce for adult self-concept. *Journal of Family Issues, 9(2)*, 75-96.

Amato, Paul R. (1986). Marital conflict, the parent-child relationship and child self esteem. *Family Relations, 35*, 403 410.

Amato, Paul R. & Ochiltree, Gay. (1987). Child and adolescent competence in intact, one-parent and step-families: an Australian study. *Journal of Divorce, 10(3-4)*, 75-96.

Amato, Paul R. & Ochiltree, Gay. (1986). Family resources and child competence. *Journal of Marriage and the Family, 48*, 47-56.

Berg, Berthold & Kelly, Robert. (1979). The measured self-esteem of children from broken, rejected and accepted families. *Journal of Divorce, 2(4)*, 363-369.

Bishop, Sue Marquis & Ingersoll, Gary M. (1989). Effects of marital conflict on the self-concepts of pre- and early adolescents. *Journal of Youth and Adolescence, 18(1)*, 25-38.

Buri, John R., Kirchner, Peggy A. & Walsh, Jane M. (1987). Familial correlates of self-esteem in young American adults. *The Journal of Social Psychology, 127(6)*, 583-588.

Burt, Charles E., Cohen, Lawrence H. & Bjork, Jeffrey P. (1988). Perceived family environment as a moderator of young adolescents' life stress adjustment. *American Journal of Community Psychology, 16(1)*, 101-122.

Cooper, Judith E., Holman, Jaqueline & Braithwaite, Valerie A. (1983). Self-esteem and family cohesion the child's perspective and adjustment. *Journal of Marriage and the Family, 45*, 153-159.

Copeland, Ann P. (1985). Individual differences in children's reaction to divorce. *Journal of Clinical Child Psychology, 14(1)*, 11-19.

Emery, Robert E. (1982). Interparental conflict and the children of discord and divorce. *Psychological Bulletin, 92(9)*, 310-330.

Geotting, Ann. (1981). Divorce outcome research issues and perspectives. *Journal of Family Issues, 2(3)*, 355-377.

Greene, Robert M. & Leslie, Leigh A. (1988). Mothers' behavior and sons' adjustment following divorce. *Journal of Divorce, 12(2-3)*, 235-251.

Hoelter, Jon & Harper, Lynn. (1987). Structural and interpersonal family influences on adolescents' self-conception. *Journal of Marriage and the Family, 49(1)*, 129-139.

Holman, Thomas, B. & Woodroofe-Patrick, Marion. (1988). Family structure, Conflict, and Children's Self-Esteem in Trinidad and Tobago. *Journal of Family Issues, 9(2)*, 214-223.

Johnson, Melanie K. & Hutchinson, Roger L. (1988). Effects of family structure on children's self-concepts. *Journal of Divorce, 12(2-3)*, 129-138.

Kanoy, Korrel W., Cunningham, Jo Lynn, White, Priscilla & Adams, Suzzane J. (1985). Is structure that critical? family relationships of children with divorced and married parents. *Journal of Divorce, 8(2)*, 97-105.

Kline, Marsha, Johnston, Janet R., and Tschann, Jeanne M. (1991). The Long Shadow of Marital Conflict: A Model of Children's Postdivorce Adjustment. *Journal of Marriage and the Family, 53*, 297-309.

Long, Barbara. (1986). Parental discord vs. family structure: effects of divorce on the self-esteem of daughters. *Journal of Youth and Adolescence, 15(1)*, 19-27.

Moos, R., & Moos, B. (1981). *Family Environment Scale Manual*. Palo Alto: Consulting Psychologist Press.

Peck, Judith Stern. (1989). The impact of divorce on children at various stages of the family life cycle. *Journal of Divorce, 12(2-3)*, 81-105.

Parish, Thomas S. (1981). Young adults evaluations of themselves and their parents as a function of family structure and disposition. *Journal of Youth and Adolescence, 10(2),* 173-178.

Partridge, Sonia & Kolter, Tamara. (1987). Self-esteem and adjustment in adolescents from bereaved, divorced, and intact families: family type versus family environment. *Australian Journal of Psychology, 39(2),* 223-234.

Stolberg, Arnold L. & Bush, Joseph P. (1985). A path analysis of factors predicting children's divorce adjustment. *Journal of Clinical Child Psychology, 14(1),* 49-54.

Swartzberg, Linda, Shmulker, Diana & Chalmers, Beverly. (1983). Emotional adjustment and self-concept of children from divorced and non-divorced unhappy homes. *The Journal of Social Psychology, 121,* 305-312.

Wallerstein, Judith S. & Blakeslee, Sandra. (1989). *Second chances Men, Women & Children of divorce who wins, who loses-and why.* New York: Ticknor & Fields.

Wiehe, Vernon. (1984). Self-esteem, attitude toward parents, and locus of control in children of divorced and non-divorced families. *Journal of Social Service Research, 8(1),* 17-28.

Wyman, Peter A., Cowen, Emory L., Hightower, A. Dirk & Pedro-Carroll, JoAnne L. (1985). *Journal of Clinical Child Psychology, 14(1),* 20-26.

Correlates
of Self-Esteem Among College Offspring
from Divorced Families:
A Study of Gender-Based Differences

Nancy J. Shook
Joan Jurich

SUMMARY. This research examines whether factors found to be relevant to children's adjustment following parental divorce do indeed have a significant relationship to the self-esteem of young adult college students who have experienced parental divorce during childhood or adolescence. These factors include gender, social class, age at the time of parental divorce, remarriage of the custodial mother, the amount of contact between the non-residential father and his offspring, and feelings of closeness between the non-residential father and his offspring. The results of a multiple regression analysis indicate that contact with the non-residential father has a significant impact on the self-esteem of female offspring, whereas the age at the time of parental divorce is the most significant factor contributing to the self-esteem of male offspring. Results also indicate there is no significant difference in self-esteem levels among male and female offspring from divorced families.

INTRODUCTION

The extent to which divorce affects children's adaptive development continues to attract the attention of researchers and clinicians

Nancy J. Shook, MS, is a doctoral student in the Department of Educational Studies, Purdue University, Wetherill Building, W. Lafayette, IN 47906.
Joan Jurich is Assistant Professor in the Department of Child Development and Family Studies, Purdue University.

© 1992 by The Haworth Press, Inc. All rights reserved.

alike. This interest is of theoretical and practical importance and is related to the fact that a large number of children under eighteen live in single parent families and to the predictions that this number will increase in the coming years (Glick, 1979; Glick & Lin, 1986). Demographically, the greatest proportion of these children live in female-headed households. Typically, these families suffer a dramatic decline in household income as a result of the divorce (Weiss, 1979) which, in turn, leads to a reduced standard of living. Hodges, Wechler, and Ballantine (1979) report that limited financial resources may be predictive of maladjustment for children of divorce. In addition, the inherently distressful process of divorce alters family interactional patterns (Hess & Camara, 1979) and may induce a crisis-like environment for all family members until the family can reorganize into a state of psychological and social equilibrium. Not surprisingly, the impact of divorce on the psychosocial adjustment of children has become the focus of numerous research studies. Indeed, the results of several studies have concluded that parental divorce has adverse effects on children's self-esteem (Boyd, Nunn, & Parish, 1983; Parish & Dostal, 1980; Parish & Taylor, 1979; Parish & Wigle, 1985; Rosenberg, 1965; Stolberg, Camplair, Currier, & Wells, 1987).

From an extensive review of the literature, a variety of factors emerge as having an important impact on the adjustment process of children following parental divorce. These factors include gender (Guidubaldi & Perry, 1985; Hess & Camara, 1979; Hetherington, Cox, & Cox, 1979; Hodges, Buschbaum, & Tierney, 1983; Lowery & Settle, 1985; Porter & O'Leary, 1980), age of the child at the time of parental divorce (Hetherington, 1972; Hetherington, Cox, & Cox, 1981; Hetherington, Stanley-Hagan, & Anderson, 1989; Kinard & Reinherz, 1984; Lowery & Settle, 1985; Rosenberg, 1965), remarriage of the custodial mother (Grossman, Shea, & Adams, 1980; Hetherington, Cox, & Cox, 1985; Parish & Dostal, 1980; Peterson & Zill, 1986), social class (Fine, Moreland, & Schwebel, 1983; Rosenberg, 1965), the amount of contact with the non-residential father (Furstenberg, Morgan, & Allison, 1987; Jacobson, 1978; Lowenstein & Koopman, 1978; Wallerstein & Kelly, 1980; 1980b; White, Brinkerhoff, & Booth, 1985) and the feelings of closeness between the non-residential father and his offspring (Hess

& Camara, 1979; Peterson & Zill, 1986; Villwock, 1987; White, Brinkerhoff, & Booth, 1985). However, little research has examined whether the impact of these factors persists as the children reach young adulthood.

The purpose of this study is to explore the extent to which these identified factors are related to the self-esteem of young adult college students who have experienced parental divorce in childhood or adolescence. Further, this study examines whether the self-esteem levels of male and female college offspring from divorced families are different from one another.

SELF-ESTEEM

Self-esteem may be defined as the overall positive or negative attitude held by an individual toward him/herself. As Rosenberg (1965) states, "When we speak of high self-esteem . . . we shall simply mean that the individual respects himself, considers himself worthy; he does not necessarily consider himself better than others, but he definitely does not considers himself worse; he does not feel that he is the ultimate in perfection but, on the contrary, he recognizes his limitations and expects to grow and improve" (p. 31).

According to Satir (1972) self-esteem is learned within the context of the family and is not carried by family genes. Infants come into the world with no previous feelings about the self and, therefore, must rely on those around them for messages which convey approval. For the first five or six years of children's lives, messages of worthiness and unworthiness are almost exclusively derived from parents and other family members. As children grow older and begin to attend school, various other agents help children shape the attitudes that they hold about themselves. These forces tend to reinforce the feelings of worthiness and unworthiness that were initially developed within the home environment. The effect of parents and family continue to influence significantly the self-esteem of children even during adolescence (Satir, 1972). The disruption of the marital bond during childhood or adolescence might then produce feelings of worthlessness or lower self-esteem in offspring because of the emotional unavailability of a parent or parents following divorce.

FACTORS EFFECTING SELF-ESTEEM

In reviewing the divorce literature, several factors are identified as effecting the development of self-esteem. These factors include gender, age at the time of parental divorce, social class, feelings of closeness in the father-offspring relationship, remarriage of the custodial mother, and frequency of contact between the non-residential father and his offspring.

Research suggests that children of various developmental ages differ qualitatively and quantitatively in their responses to parental divorce (Hetherinton, Stanley-Hagan, & Anderson, 1989; Wallerstein & Kelly, 1976). Several studies have found that children who are six years old or younger at the time of parental divorce, as compared to those who are older than six years, are less likely to experience a favorable post-divorce adjustment (Gardner, 1976; Hetherington, 1972; McDermott, 1968; Rosenberg, 1965). Younger children are more cognitively immature than older children and do not have the ability to construct either concrete or abstract adaptive resolutions to problems. Rather, young children resort to more primitive coping strategies such as fantasy and denial to manage their losses. Thus, the cognitive maturity of older children and adolescents allows them to assess more accurately the role that their parents play in the divorce situation. In addition, adolescents and young adults are likely to have access to social support networks and mental health services, improving their chances to cope with psychological and behavioral problems which are related to parental divorce (Farber, Primavera, & Felner, 1983). In light of this knowledge, age at the time of parental divorce becomes a variable which warrants attention when assessing self-esteem levels of divorced offspring.

An association between social class and self-esteem was established in several studies (Demo & Savin-Williams, 1983; Rosenberg, 1965; Rosenberg & Pearlin, 1978). The consistent results of these studies reveal that a positive relationship exists between social class and self-esteem of individuals of various different ages. Moreover, it appears that social class becomes a stronger determinant of self-esteem as people age. Therefore, it is conceivable that families with high annual incomes can offer their children more privileges than families who report more meager family incomes. This freedom provides children with the opportunities to achieve social competency and personal goals which lead to high self-esteem. Thus, there seems to be evidence to suggest that social class may also be relevant to the study of self-esteem among college offspring from divorced families.

There is a controversy over whether or not the presence of a step-father influences post-divorce adjustment in offspring. Some studies suggest that the self-esteem of offspring from mother-re-married families and mother-not-remarried families do not differ (Parish & Dostal, 1980; Parish & Taylor, 1979; Young & Parish, 1977). However, other studies suggest that offspring whose divorced mothers remarry adjust more favorably to parental divorce (Hetherington et al., 1985; Oshman & Manosevitz, 1976; Peterson & Zill, 1986). Still other studies indicate that there is a negative relationship between remarriage of the custodial mother and children's self-esteem (Rosenberg, 1965; Thies, 1977). In light of this discrepancy in findings and the possible importance of remarriage to children's self-esteem, this variable was included in the present study to examine its contribution to the development of self-esteem in young adult college offspring.

Contact between the non-residential father and his offspring also has a profound affect on the adjustment process of children of divorce. Although some research shows that contact with non-custodial fathers is unrelated to behavioral measures of children's well-being (Furstenberg, Morgan, & Allison, 1987), there is much evidence to support the notion that children who have less frequent contact with their non-residential fathers have more negative attitudes towards themselves (Guidubaldi & Perry, 1986; Jacobson, 1978; Kurdek & Berg, 1983; Lowenstein & Koopman, 1978; Wallerstein & Kelly, 1980). Contact can provide children with the reassurance that the departed parent still cares for his offspring (Wallerstein & Kelly, 1980) as well as strengthen the relationship between the non-residential father and his offspring (White et al.,

1985). Thus, contact between offspring and their non-residential fathers was examined with other variables to assess its influence on the self-esteem of divorced offspring as they are reaching adulthood.

In addition to contact, closeness between non-residential father and offspring has been found to have a significant impact on the post-divorce adjustment of children (Rosenberg, 1965; Villwock, 1987; White, Brinkerhoff, & Booth, 1985). In fact, White et al. (1985) report that closeness between the non-residential father and his offspring actually increases when the custodial mother remarries and the stepfather brings his own children to the new family. Conceivably, the presence of step-siblings produces greater competition for limited parental attention. This competition might then prompt offspring to seek affection from the non-custodial father, resulting in a stronger parent-child relationship. In view of this process, closeness between the non-residential father and his offspring is examined for its contribution to self-esteem levels.

Finally, there are few studies which present with any certainty that either males or females are more adversely affected by parental divorce. In fact, some researchers suggest that males are more adversely affected (Guidubaldi & Perry, 1985; Hammond, 1979; Hess & Camara, 1979; Hetherington et al., 1979; Hodges, Buchsbaum, & Tierney, 1983; Santrock & Warshak, 1979), while others argue for the reverse effect (Hetherington, 1972; Wallerstein & Kelly, 1985). The fact that these discrepant findings occur suggests that gender may play a complex role in how children respond to parental divorce.

For example, the psychosocial adjustment of children to parental divorce may be influenced by their developmental process. This process, according to Carol Gilligan (1982), is different for male and female children. Gilligan (1982) states that males tend to forge an identity through successfully separating from their mothers and others in the outside world while females tend to develop an identity within the context of social interactions and through attachment to others. Males also tend to seek control over things which offer potential happiness and often engage in interpersonal competition to gain such objects. Alternatively, females tend to limit their aggression in order to establish a more co-operative and interdependent relationship with another. Thus, males and females may react differently to the loss of a steady relationship with the departing parent and certain aspects of the divorce process may differentially affect the emotional well-being of male and female offspring. In light of these findings, males and females were examined separately to determine whether the relationship between independent variables and self-esteem is similar among male and female offspring from divorced families.

METHODS

Sample

The research was conducted at a large midwestern university in the fall of 1988. A self-report questionnaire was administered to under-graduates who were enrolled in an introductory marriage and family relationships class. Students were enrolled in a variety of majors across all schools within the university. All of the students were volunteers, between the ages of eighteen and twenty-three years, had experienced parental divorce during childhood or adolescence, and were from families in which the mother had been awarded primary child custody and had been divorced only once.

The sample consisted of 81 respondents, 69% ($N = 56$) of whom were female and 31% ($N = 25$) of whom were male. Male students were predominantly seniors (52%, $N = 13$). The greatest percentage of females (50%, $N = 28$) in this study were sophomores. The majority (over 80%) of both males and females were Caucasian. The average age of male offspring at the time of his parents' divorce was 12.0 years (SD = 6.8) whereas the mean age of females was 9.7 years (SD = 5.8). Fifty-four percent ($N = 44$) of the students were from backgrounds in which the mother had not remarried. The remaining students were from backgrounds in which the mother had remarried. When the two groups were compared, the remarried group had experienced parental divorce at an earlier age (Mean = 8.2, SD = 5.9) than the non-remarried group (Mean = 12.4, SD = 5.9).

Instrumentation

Self-esteem was measured using the 10-item Rosenberg Self-Esteem Inventory (Rosenberg, 1965). This scale consists of 10 Likert-type statements, phrased both positively and negatively. Sample statements include "I am able to do things as well as most people" and "I certainly feel useless at times." Students were asked to indicate how strongly they agreed or disagreed with each of the ten statements according to a 4-point scale, ranging from strongly disagree (1) to strongly agree (4). Thus, self-esteem scores could range from 10 to 40 with the lowest scores reflecting low self-esteem. The Cronbach's alpha reliability coefficient for this scale was 0.87 for both the males and females in this study.

Feelings of closeness with the non-residential father were measured with seventeen questions developed by Villwock (1987). Using factor analysis, she analyzed five instruments pertaining to father-child closeness and identified a single closeness factor. Items loading .70 and above on this factor were used in the present analysis. These items address the students' feelings of closeness to their non-residential father. Sample items include "How confident are you that your father would help you when you have a problem"; "How much do you trust your father"; "How close do you feel toward your father?" Participants responded to each question on a 7- point scale ranging from "not at all" (1) to "a great deal" (7). Thus, scores could vary from 17 (very unattached to father) to 119 (very close to father). The Cronbach's alpha reliability for this measure was 0.97 for males and 0.99 for females in this sample.

Contact with the non-residential father was conceptualized as the amount of time that offspring resided with the non-custodial father over the past year. The ten response categories ranged from "not at all" (1) to "a total of 11-12 months" (10). Due to the skewed distribution of student responses, this variable was dichotomized into "no time spent" ($N = 56$) and "some time spent" ($N = 25$) with the non-custodial father.

Finally, in addition to obtaining demographic information such as gender, age at the time of parental divorce, and whether or not the custodial mother had remarried, post-divorce social class was assessed with the Two Factor Index of Social Position (Myers &

Bean, 1968). This index consists of an educational and occupational status scale. Numerical values from 1 to 7 are assigned to levels of educational and occupational achievement within each scale. Lower scores reflect higher levels of educational and occupational prestige. To compute educational scores, the assigned numerical values for achieved educational levels are multiplied by a predetermined weight of 4. Thus, educational scores can range from 4 to 28, lower scores indicating achievement of a graduate degree. Occupational scores are computed by taking the predetermined weight of 7 and multiplying it with the numerical value assigned to a particular occupational category. Occupational scores can vary from 7 to 49, lower scores indicating greater occupational prestige. For the post-divorced, not-remarried family, social class is based on the summed educational and occupational prestige scores of the divorced mother. For the post-divorced, remarried family, social class is based on the average of the mothers' and stepfathers' combined educational and occupational prestige scores. Post-divorce social class scores can vary from 11 (very high socio-economic status) to 77 (very low socio-economic status).

RESULTS

When the data from the female group were subjected to correlational analysis, the correlations among the independent variables were low to moderate (see Table 1).

In light of the magnitude of these correlations, collinearity was not likely to be a problem in the regression analysis for females. A standard multiple regression was conducted with age at the time of parental divorce, remarriage of the custodial mother, social class of the post-divorce family, contact with the non-residential father, and feelings of closeness for the non-residential father as the independent variables and self-esteem scores as the dependent variable. Since neither theory nor previous research suggests an order of importance, all of the variables were entered simultaneously into the equation rather than entering the variables in a specified order. The results of the multiple regression analysis for self-esteem among female college offspring are presented in Table 2.

Table 1

Bivariate Pearsonian Correlations of Variables Used in the Female Model
Analyses

	AF	CO	SES	REM	AGE
SE	.01	-.31	.22	.07	.06
AF		.58	-.05	-.05	.27
CO			.16	-.12	.08
SES				.16	.20
REM					.32

Note. SE = self-esteem; AF = feelings of closeness for the non-resdential
father; CO = contact with the non-residential father as measured by the
amount of time that offspring have resided with their fathers over the
past year; SES = social class of the post-divorce family; REM = remarriage
of the custodial mother; AGE = age of offspring at the time of parental
divorce.

N = 56.

The combination of independent variables produced an adjusted
R-square of 0.08 for female self-esteem, indicating that about eight
percent of the variance in female self-esteem was accounted for by
the five predictors in the equation. However, this contribution was
not significant: $[F(5,50) = 1.98$, N. S.].

Upon closer inspection of the results, contact with the non-residential father had the strongest association with female self-esteem
(Beta = -0.43, $p < .01$; unique contribution = .12). Contrary to
expectation, greater contact between female offspring and their
non-residential fathers is associated with lower self-esteem among
female offspring from divorced families. Feelings of closeness for
the non-residential father has the next strongest relationship with
female self-esteem (Beta = .25; $p = .14$, N.S.) and suggests that
greater feelings of closeness for the non-residential father is

Table 2

Standard Multiple Regression of Independent Variables on Self-Esteem of
Female College Offspring from Divorced Families

	Unstandardized Beta	Beta		sr-square
AGE	-0.00	-.00		.00
CO	-1.18	-.43		.12 **
SES	.05	.13		.02
REM	.10	.01		.00
AF	.03	.25		.04
Multiple R			.41	
F(5, 50)			1.98	
Adjusted R-square			.08	

Note. AGE = age of offspring at the time of parental divorce; CO = contact
with the non-residential father as measured by the amount of time that
offspring resided with their fathers over the past year; SES = social class
of the post-divorce family; REM = remarriage of the custodial mother;
AF = feelings of closeness for the non-residential father.

Intercept = 34.65.

sr-square = unique contribution of independent variable.

** $p < .01$.

N = 56.

associated with higher self-esteem in female offspring. However,
this finding was not statistically significant.

The data from the male sample also was subjected to correlational and standard multiple regression analysis. Results of the correlational analysis are displayed in Table 3.

Again, due to low to moderate correlations among independent
variables, collinearity was not a problem (see Table 4).

In contrast to the female model, the results of the multiple regres-

Table 3

Bivariate Pearsonian Correlations of Variables Used in the Male Model
Analyses

	AF	CO	SES	REM	AGE
SE	-.09	-.16	.33	.17	.49
AF		.57	.34	.45	.46
CO			.25	.39	.15
SES				.30	.43
REM					.36

Note. SE = self-esteem; AF = feelings of closeness for the non-
residential father; CO = contact with the non-residential father as
measured by the amount of time that offspring have resided with their
father over the past year; REM = remarriage of the custodial mother;
AGE = age of offspring at the time of parental divorce.
N= 25.

sion analysis among male offspring were found to be significantly
different from zero: [F(5,19) = 2.86, p < .05].

The combination of the independent variables produced an adjusted R-square of .28 for male offspring, indicating that 28% of the variance in self-esteem among male offspring from divorced families was accounted for by the predictor variables. The variable most strongly related to self-esteem was age of the child at the time of parental divorce (Beta = 0.56, p < .05, unique contribution = .20). The older the male offspring was at the time of divorce, the greater was his level of self-esteem. As with the females, feelings of closeness to the non-residential father had the next strongest relationship with self-esteem (Beta = −.41, p = .10, N. S.). Contrary to expectation, closeness to father is associated with lower self-esteem. However, the finding was not statistically significant.

In addition to the regression analysis, a 2 (gender) × 2 (family structure) analysis of variance with self-esteem as the dependent

Table 4

Standardized Multiple Regression of the Independent Varaibles on Self-
Esteem of Male College Offspring from Divorced Families

	Unstandardized Beta	Beta		sr-square
AGE	0.39	.56		.20 *
CO	-0.33	-.12		.01
SES	.08	.22		.04
REM	1.25	.14		.01
AF	-0.07	-.42		.09
Multiple R			.66	
F (5, 19)			2.86 *	
Adjusted R-square			.28	

Note. AGE = age of offspring at the time of parental divorce; CO = contact with the non-residential father as measured by the amount of time that offspring have rsided with their fathers over the past year; SES = social class of the post divorce family; REM = remarriage of the custodial father; AF = feelings of closeness for the non-residential father.

Intercept = 33.71.

sr-square = unique contribution of independent variables.

* $p < .05$.

N= 25.

variable was conducted to examine whether offspring self-esteem varies with family structure (remarried vs. non-remarried) and gender (male vs. female). The results indicated that offspring from remarried families (Mean = 31.78, SD = 4.42) and non-remarried families (Mean = 32.66, SD = 4.67) do not differ from one another [F (1,77) = 7.66, p = .38, N. S.] and that male offspring from divorced families (Mean = 32.04, SD = 4.61) do not differ from females (Mean = 32.36, SD = 4.57) in self-esteem levels [F(1,77) = 1.24, p = .73, N. S.]. In addition, there was no interactional effect [F(1,77) = 1.78, p = .67, N.S.]. That is, males and females from remarried and non-remarried families do not differ on self-esteem ratings.

A group of students from the same class but from intact families was also examined for self-esteem. The mean self-esteem scores for males of this group was 32.34 (SD = 4.05). The average female score was 31.08 (SD = 4.13). When compared to their classmates, offspring from divorced backgrounds do not appear to rate themselves much differently on levels of self- esteem. In fact, college offspring from divorced families appear to rate themselves fairly high when considering that the highest possible score on the Rosenberg Scale is 40.

DISCUSSION

When separate regressions were performed on the male and female offspring groups, the findings supported Gilligan's notion that separate factors account for the characteristic ways in which males and females define themselves. The results of the female regression analysis suggest that contact with the non-residential father had a significant but negative impact on self-esteem scores, whereas age at the time of parental divorce emerged as a significant and positive predictor of male but not female self-esteem ratings. Thus, it appears that the longer male offspring are exposed to the positive influence of their fathers, the greater their self-esteem. By contrast, early father absence does not appear to significantly affect female self-esteem. Perhaps, the quality of the mother-daughter relationship resulting from same-sex custody (Santrock and Warshak, 1979) buffers any adverse effects which may result from the loss of the opposite-gender parent.

Findings about the direction of the relationship between female offspring self-esteem and contact with the non-residential fathers were contrary to expectation. However, the negative relationship is plausible according to family therapists, Bepko & Krestan (1990). According to these authors, females are socialized to be unselfish, to focus on the happiness of others, and to place the needs of others above their own in order to feel valued, loved, or competent. Thus, when females subscribe to external guidelines about how they should behave, they are at risk for feeling vulnerable to the opinions of others about their worthiness. Perhaps, female offspring with greater contact with non-residential fathers spend their time focusing on meeting the needs and expectations of their fathers. In offering this time and attention, female offspring may assume responsibility for their fathers' happiness and comfort and become overconcerned with their fathers' reactions to them. Failure to gain the approval of their fathers may lead female offspring to report low levels of self-esteem.

Data from this study did not, however, support the idea that the presence of a stepfather could be beneficial for divorced offspring (Oshman and Manosevitz, 1976). Rather, the findings of this study suggest that the remarriage of the custodial mother neither detracts nor enhances self-esteem ratings of offspring from divorced families. Perhaps, it is the quality of the relationship between the stepfather and his offspring rather than the absence or presence of a father figure that influences the self-esteem of offspring from remarried families. Another possibility may be that offspring from non-remarried families grew up in households with mothers who were well-educated and had occupations with economic security. In fact, results of this study show that 50% ($N = 22$) of the mothers who did not remarry had achieved either a bachelor or graduate college degree, while only 27% ($N = 10$) of mothers who remarried achieved a similar education. Likewise, the findings reveal that 40.9% ($N = 18$) of non-remarried mothers had executive, managerial, or administrative positions, while only 25% ($N = 9$) of the remarried mothers held managerial or administrative positions. Thus, the financial advantage associated with the occupational and educational prestige of the non-remarried mother may act as a protective factor which insulates offspring against the potential psychological distress due to the loss of a biological parent.

Moreover, the results of this study do not support the notion that being six years old or younger at the onset of parental divorce potentially increases the children's risk for a less favorable post-divorce adjustment. More specifically, when the self-esteem scores of those who had experienced parental divorce after the age of six (Mean = 32.35, SD = 4.62, N = 51) were compared with those who had experienced parental divorce at the age of six or younger (Mean = 32.04, SD = 4.67, N = 28), the latter group did not demonstrate significantly lower self-esteem scores (t = −.29, p = .77, NS). Conceivably, the long-term outcome of those offspring who were younger at the time of their parents' divorce and who became college students have had access to economic resources and social networks which have allowed them to overcome difficulties associated with their parents' divorce.

Finally, the findings of this study are consistent with those of other researchers who report that parental divorce does not adversely affect the average, overall level of self-esteem of offspring (Berg & Kelly, 1979; Gabardi & Rosén, 1991; Hammond, 1979; Parish, 1981; Raschke & Raschke, 1979; Wyman, Cowen, Hightower, & Pedro-Carroll, 1985). The fact that offspring from divorced families appear to rate themselves similarly to their classmates from intact families suggests that family structure does not predispose individuals to lower levels of self-esteem. In fact, females from divorced families actually rate themselves higher in self-esteem (Mean = 32.36, SD = 4.57) than their female counterparts from intact families (Mean = 31.08, SD = 4.13). Moreover, males from divorced families report just slightly lower (Mean = 32.04, SD = 4.61) self-esteem ratings than those males from intact families (Mean = 32.34, SD = 4.05).

The findings of this study should be viewed with caution because the sample of college students surveyed in this study may not be representative of college students elsewhere or to non-college samples. Therefore, findings in this study may not be generalized to other populations. Also, the size of the sample under investigation was small and failure to find more statistically significant findings may have resulted. Finally, data was collected through self-reports and therefore, social desirability may have been a problem. These methodological limitations can be addressed in future research by increasing the sample sizes under investigation, using behavioral and observational assessments to corroborate findings, and using samples which include offspring from a greater diversity of educational backgrounds.

CONCLUSION

In sum, the proposed regression explained a higher percentage of variance in male than female self-esteem with only the male model demonstrating statistical significance. Therefore, further research might focus on identifying additional factors which influence the females' psychosocial adjustment to parental divorce. Likewise, further research is warranted if other key factors in the adjustment process of male offspring from divorced families are to be identified.

REFERENCES

Bepko, C. & Krestan, J. (1990). *Too good for her own good: Searching for self and intimacy in important relationships.* New York, NY: Harper and Row, Pub., Inc.

Berg, B. & Kelly, R. (1979). The measured self-esteem of children from broken, rejected, and accepted families. *Journal of Divorce, 2*, 363-370.

Boyd, D., Nunn, G. & Parish, T. (1983). Effects of marital status on evaluations of self and parents. *Journal of Social Psychology, 119*, 229-234.

Bumpass, L. & Rindfuss, R. (1979). Children's experience of marital disruption. *American Journal of Sociology, 85*, 49-65.

Demo, D. H. & Savin-Williams, R. C. (1983). Early-adolescent self-esteem as a function of social class: Rosenberg and Pearlin revisited. *American Journal of Sociology, 88*, 763-774.

Farber, S. S., Primavera, J., & Felner, R. D. (1983). Older adolescents and parental divorce: Adjustment problems and mediators of coping. *Journal of Divorce, 7*, 59-75.

Fine, M. A., Moreland, J. R., & Schwebel, A. I. (1983). Long-term effects of divorce on parent-child relationships. *Developmental Psychology, 19*, 703-713.

Furstenberg, F. F., Morgan, S. P., & Allison, P. D. (1987). Paternal participation and children's well-being after marital dissolution. *American Sociological Review, 52*, 695-701.

Gabardi, L. & Rosén, L. A. (1991). Differences between college students from divorced and intact families. *Journal of Divorce and Remarriage, 15*, 175-191.

Gardner, R. (1976). *Psychotherapy with children of divorce.* New York, New York: Jason Aronson, Inc.

Gilligan, C. (1982). *In a different voice: Psychological theory and women's development.* Cambridge, MA: Havard University Press.

Glick, P. C. (1979). Children of divorced parents in demographic perspective. *Journal of Social Issues, 35*, 170-182.

174   *DIVORCE AND THE NEXT GENERATION*

Glick, P. C. & Lin, S. L. (1986). Recent changes in divorce and remarriage. *Journal of Marriage and the Family, 48,* 737-747.

Guidubaldi, J., & Perry, J. (1985). Divorce and the mental health sequelae for children: A two year follow-up of a nationwide sample. *Journal of the American Academy of Child Psychiatry, 24,* 531-537.

Grossman, S. M., Shea, J. A., & Adams, G. R. (1980). Effects of parental divorce during early childhood on ego development and identity formation of college students. *Journal of Divorce, 3,* 263-272.

Hammond, J. (1979). Children of divorce: A study of self-concept, academic achievement, and attitudes. *The Elementary School Journal, 80,* 55-62.

Hess, R., & Camara, K. (1979). Post-divorce relationships as mediating factors in the consequences of divorce for children. *Journal of Social Issues, 35,* 75-95.

Hetherington, E. M. (1972). Effects of paternal absence on personality development in adolescent daughters. *Developmental Psychology, 7,* 313-326.

Hetherington, E. M., Cox, M., & Cox, R. (1979). Play and the social interaction in children following divorce. *Journal of Social Issues, 35,* 26-49.

Hetherington, E. M., Cox, M., & Cox, R. (1981). The aftermath of divorce. In *Contemporary readings in child psychology* (2nd Ed.). New York: McGraw-Hill Inc.

Hetherington, E. M., Cox, M., & Cox, R. (1985). Long-term effects of divorce and remarriage on the adjustment of children. *Journal of the Academy of Child Psychiatry, 24,* 518-530.

Hetherington, Stanley-Hagan, M., & Anderson, E. R. (1989). Marital transitions: A child's perspective. *American Psychologist, 44,* 303- 312.

Hodges, W. F., Buchsbaum, R. C., & Tierney, C. W. (1983). Parent-child relationships and adjustment in preschool children in divorced and intact families. *Journal of Divorce, 7,* 43-58.

Hodges, W. F., Wechsler, R. C., & Ballantine, C. (1979). Divorce and the preschool child: Cumulative stress. *Journal of Divorce, 3,* 55-67.

Jacobson, D. S. (1978). The impact of marital separation/divorce on children: 1. Parent-child separation and child adjustment. *Journal of Divorce, 1,* 341-357.

Kinard, E. M. & Reinherz, H. (1984). Marital disruption: Effects on behavioral and emotional functioning in children. *Journal of Family Issues, 5,* 90-115.

Kurdeck, L. A. & Berg, B. (1983). Correlates of children's adjustment to their parents' divorce. in L. A. Kurdek (Ed.), *Children and divorce* (pp. 47- 60). San Francisco: Jossey-Bass Inc., Publishers.

Lowenstein, J. & Koopmn, E. (1978). A comparison of the self-esteem between boys living with single-parent mothers and single parent fathers. *Journal of Divorce, 2,* 195-208.

Lowery, C. R. & Settle, S. A. (1985). Effects of divorce on children: Differential impact of custody and visitation pattern. *Family Relations, 34,* 455-463.

McDermott, J. (1968). Parental divorce in early childhood. *American Journal of Psychiatry, 124,* 1424-1434.

Myers, J. K. & Bean, L. L. (1968). *A decade later: A follow-up of social class and mental illness.* New York: John Wiley & Sons, Inc.

Oshman, H. & Manosevitz, M. (1976). Father absence: Effects of stepfathers upon the psychosocial development in males. *Developmental Psychology, 12,* 479-480.

Parish, T. (1981). The impact of divorce on the family. *Adolescence, 16,* 577-580.

Parish, T. & Dostal, J. (1980). Evaluations of self and parent figures by children from intact, divorced, and reconstituted families. *Journal of Youth and Adolescence, 9,* 347-351.

Parish T. & Taylor, J. (1979). The impact of divorce and subsequent father absence on children's and adolescents' self-concepts. *Journal of Youth and Adolescence, 8,* 427-432.

Parish T. & Wigle, S. (1985). A longitudinal study of the impact of parental divorce on adolescents' evaluation of self and parents. *Adolescence, 77,* 239-244.

Peterson, J. L. & Zill, N. (1986). Marital disruption, parent-child relationships, and behavioral problems in children. *Journal of Marriage and the Family, 48,* 295-307.

Porter, B. & O'Leary, K. D. (1980). Marital discord and childhood behavior problems. *Journal of Abnormal Child Psychology, 8,* 287-295.

Raschke, H. & Raschke, V. (1979). Family conflict and children's self-concepts: A comparison of intact and single parent families. *Journal of Marriage and the Family, 41,* 367-374.

Rosenberg, M. (1965). *Society and the adolescent self-image.* New Jersey: Princeton University Press.

Rosenberg, F. R. & Pearlin, L. I. (1978). Social class and self-esteem among children and adults. *American Journal of Sociology, 84,* 53-77.

Santrock, J. & Warshak, R. (1979). Father custody and social development in boys and girls. *Journal of Social Issues, 35,* 112-125.

Satir, V. (1972). *Peoplemaking.* Palo Alto, CA: Science and Behavior Books, Inc.

Stolberg, A. L., Camplair, C., Currier, K., & Wells, M. J. (1987). Individual, familial and environmental determinants of children's post-divorce adjustment and maladjustment. *Journal of Divorce, 11,* 51-70.

Thies, J. (1977). Beyond divorce: The impact of remarriage on children. *Journal of Clinical Child Psychology, 6,* 59-61.

Villwock, D. (1987). *Closeness in father-offspring relationships: Do differences linked to parental marital status persist in a multivariate approach?* Unpublished doctoral dissertation, Purdue University, West Lafayette, IN.

Wallerstein, J. S. (1985). Children of divorce: Preliminary report of a ten-year follow-up of older children and adolescents. *Journal of the American Academy of Child Psychiatry, 24,* 545-553.

Wallerstein, J. S. (1987). Children of divorce: Report of a ten-year follow-up of early latency-age children. *American Journal of Orthopsychiatry, 57,* 199-211.

Wallerstein, J. S. & Kelly, J. B. (1980). Effects of divorce on the visiting father-child relationship. *American Journal of Psychiatry, 137,* 1534-1539.

Wallerstein, J. S. & Kelly, J. B. (1980b). *Surviving the breakup: How children and parents cope with divorce.* New York: Basic Books, Inc.

Weiss, Robert. (1979). Growing up a little faster: The experiences of growing up in a single-parent household. *Journal of Social Issues*, 35, 97-111.

White, L. K., Brinkerhoff, D. B., & Booth, A. (1985). Effects of marital disruption on children's attachment to parents. *Journal of Family Issues*, 6, 5-22.

Wyman, P. A., Cowen, E. L., Hightower, A. D., & Pedro-Carrol, J. L. (1985). Perceived competency, self-esteem, and anxiety in the latency-aged children of divorce. *Journal of Clinical Child Psychology*, 14, 217-226.

Selected Aspects of Parenting and Children's Social Competence Post-Separation: The Moderating Effects of Child's Sex, Age, and Family Economic Hardship

Cheryl Buehler
Bobbie H. Legg

SUMMARY. The purpose of this study was to assess the moderating effects of child's sex, ace, and family economic hardship on the relationship between (a) residential mother's parenting and frequency of nonresidential father's visitation, and (b) child social competence following marital separation. Dimensions of mother's parenting included loss of time spent with the child since separation, mother's current levels of companionship and coercion, and daily involvement in meaningful activities with the child. Dimensions of children's social competence included dependency, aggression, anxiety/withdrawal, and productivity. The results indicated that the relationships among mother's parenting, father's visitation, and children's social competence are fairly consistent, regardless of child's age, sex, or

---

Cheryl Buehler, PhD, is Associate Professor in the Department of Child and Family Studies, JHB 115, University of Tennessee, Knoxville, TN 37996. Bobbie Legg, PhD, is Coordinator at East Tennessee Comprehensive Hemophilia Center, Knoxville, TN 37996.

The authors would like to thank Phyllis Betz, Bill Swann, and the late Mary Evans for their professional support of this project, and Catherine Ryan and Belinda Trotter for their assistance in data collection. The study reported in this paper was supported partially by a Faculty Research Award to the second author from the University of Tennessee-Knoxville.

© 1992 by The Haworth Press, Inc. All rights reserved.

level of family economic hardship. The few exceptions are noted and intervention implications are discussed.

Between now and the end of the twentieth century, 33% of this generation of children will experience parental divorce before they are 18 (Glick, 1984). Although divorce does not invariably result in enduring adverse outcomes for children, the process does entail a series of stressful experiences (Hetherington & Camara, 1984). Children are particularly vulnerable to adjustment problems when parent-child relationships are seriously disrupted or are of generally poor quality (Hetherington, 1989; Kurdek, 1987; Peterson & Zill, 1986; Tschann, Johnston, Kline, & Wallerstein, 1989; Wallerstein, Corbin, & Lewis, 1988). There also is some evidence that children's vulnerability postseparation varies with their age (Allison & Furstenberg, 1989; Kurdek & Berg, 1983; Tschann, Johnston, Kline, & Wallerstein, 1990; Wallerstein et al., 1988), by sex (Block, Block, & Gjerde, 1986; Hetherington, Cox, & Cox, 1982; Peterson & Zill, 1986; Tschann et al., 1990), and with family economic hardship (Ambert, 1984; Colletta, 1983; Guidubaldi & Perry, 1985).

It is unclear, however, whether children's age, sex, and family economic well-being moderate the relationship between parent-child relationships and children's social competence following marital separation or effect competence only directly. The examination of moderating effects is very different from that of direct effects. A variable exhibiting direct effects influences the level of a dependent variable, whereas a moderating variable changes either the strength or direction of a *relationship between variables* (James & Brett, 1984). For example, the question of whether or not boys are more aggressive than girls postseparation involves testing the *direct effect* of sex of child on aggressive behavior. Very differently, the question of whether or not the relationship between mother's coercive parenting and child aggression is different for boys and girls involves testing the *moderating* effect of sex of child on the *relationship between* mother's coercion and child aggression. Therefore, the purpose of this study was to examine the moderating effects of child sex, age, and family economic hardship on the relationships between (a) several indicators of mothers' reports of her parenting and children's social competence (CSC) post-separation, and (b) mothers' reports of frequency of father visitation and CSC post-separation. The focus was on residential mothers and nonresidential fathers because mothers continue to receive custody of children in 90% of divorced families (Furstenberg & Nord, 1985).

This study makes several contributions to the research on children's adjustment to parental separation. First, both parenting and CSC are conceptualized as multidimensional constructs. Kurdek (1987) has illustrated the importance of examining multidimensional conceptualizations. Second, the moderating effects of the child's age, sex, and economic well-being are assessed. The moderating effects of these variables on the relationship between parental involvement and CSC have not been examined systematically in previous research on children's adjustment postseparation. Addressing potential moderators is important because researchers have begun to acknowledge "that the influence of parent-child relations on child development" is not the same across all children (Belsky, 1990, p. 889). The significance or nonsignificance of key moderators will influence the specifics of parenting information integrated into various divorce prevention and intervention programs. Finally, a nonclinical sample drawn from court records is used to generate results that can be used validly to develop community-based programs.

LITERATURE REVIEW

Sex of Child

Several researchers have examined the *direct effects* of child's sex on CSC postseparation. Three general conclusions can be drawn from these tests. First, sons have more short-term adjustment problems postdivorce (1-2 years) than do daughters (Demo & Acock, 1988; Hetherington & Camara, 1984; Wallerstein et al., 1988). Second, this pattern is strongest when undercontrolled, externalized child behaviors are examined (e.g., aggression, conduct disorders) rather than overcontrolled, internalized behaviors (e.g., withdrawal)(Dadds, 1987; Demo & Acock, 1988; Patterson, DeBaryshe, & Ramsey, 1989). Third, although these conclusions have been supported using data from various and numerous samples of children, some scholars using national data have not found sex differences (Allison & Furstenberg, 1989; Zaslow, 1987).

Although scholars have suggested that poor and differential maternal parenting, and disrupted father involvement are two of the reasons sons may have a more difficult time adjusting to marital separation than do daughters (Emery, Hetherington, & DiLalla, 1984), the interaction analyses that would support these explanations have not been conducted. It has been suggested in discussions of the research conducted by Hetherington and her colleagues (Emery et al., 1984; Hetherington, 1989; Hetherington & Camara, 1981; Hetherington et al., 1982) that the relationship between mother's parenting and CSC is stronger for boys than girls. However, it is not clear from these discussions how the interaction terms between sex of child and mother's parenting variables were tested. Description of the statistical tests used states that "multivariate analyses, followed by univariate analysis of significant multivariate effects, with sex of child and family types as the independent measures were performed on the composite indices of parent and child behaviors" (Hetherington, 1987, p. 191). Thus, although their research may suggest moderating effects (particularly for younger children), it is not clear that these effects were tested explicitly.

Other scholars have suggested moderating effects for sex of child by analyzing the relationship between parenting variables and dimensions of CSC separately for sons and daughters. Using this type of analysis, Peterson and Zill (1986) reported differences in patterns and magnitudes of correlations that may suggest possible moderating effects.

Thus, although moderating effects of sex of child on the relationship between parenting and CSC postseparation have not been tested directly, indirect evidence suggests that the relationship may be stronger for sons than daughters, particularly when externalized indices of CSC are examined. This hypothesis was tested in the present study.

Age of Child

The direct effects of child's age on social competence post-separation are unclear, inconsistent, and poorly researched (Emery,

1982; Emery et al., 1984). Some researchers have found that younger children have more difficulties than older ones (Allison & Furstenberg, 1989; Kurdek & Berg, 1983; Wallerstein et al., 1988), whereas others have found the opposite (Tschann et al., 1990). Rather than conceptualize the effects of child age as linear, some scholars have suggested that children ages six to eleven (middle school-age) have a more difficult time adjusting than either younger children or adolescents (Camara & Resnick, 1988; Guidubaldi, Cleminshaw, Perry, & Kehle, 1983; Jacobson, 1978; Kalter & Rembar, 1981).

However, because none of these researchers reported calculating age by parenting interaction terms, the moderating effects of age of child are unknown. Thus, one of the purposes of this study was to examine the moderating effects of age on the relationship between parenting and CSC postseparation. Using suggestions from extant findings and Erikson's (1968) development of the major social-emotional tasks during the middle years of childhood, it was hypothesized, that the relationship between parenting and CSC would be stronger for children ages six to eleven than for children of other ages.

Family Economic Hardship

Research conducted by Guidubaldi and associates indicates that many of the differences in social competence between children from divorced and nondivorced families disappear when family income is controlled (Guidubaldi & Perry, 1984, 1985). However, the moderating effect of economic hardship on the relationship between parenting and CSC has not been examined empirically. Although few scholars have discussed possible moderating effects, for this study it was hypothesized that the relationship between mothers' parenting and CSC would be stronger for those children whose mothers perceived themselves as struggling economically than for those children whose mothers perceived themselves as economically stable. The rationale for this hypothesis was based on the idea that effective and nondisruptive parenting would be more salient under conditions of economic hardship than economic stability. This rationale is similar to that used by Shaw and Emery

(1988) when they argued that factors such as concurrent poor parenting and economic hardships pile-up, increasing children's vulnerability.

Control Variables

Recent reviews of literature on children's social competence following marital separation suggest several important control variables: parent's age, education, months from separation, and parental conflict (Demo & Acock, 1988; Hetherington & Camara, 1984). These variables were included in the present study as controls. Perhaps more importantly, researchers have shown that mothers' psychosocial well-being (e.g., depression) is correlated moderately with their reports of CSC (Belsky, 1990; Brody & Forehand, 1988; Forgatch, Patterson, & Skinner, 1988; Furstenberg & Seltzer, 1986; Guidubaldi & Perry, 1985; Shaw & Emery, 1988) and with child reports of CSC (Furstenberg & Seltzer, 1986; Kurdek & Berg, 1983). These correlations seem to be due to shared systematic variance (about two-thirds) and shared agent variance (about one-third). Thus, mother's well-being must be controlled for when examining the relationship between mother's reports of parenting and CSC.

METHODS

Research Design and Sampling

A sample of 108 divorcing mothers was obtained from court records in a fairly large southeastern community. Couples who had filed for divorce in 1986 were sampled. Because this study was part of a larger project, a rather lengthy questionnaire was mailed to all potential participants. Up to three mail contacts were attempted with most subjects in the sampling frame. Questionnaires were sent to 422 separated mothers. Of these 422, 79 (19%) of the questionnaires were nondeliverable and 148 of the mothers completed and returned questionnaires (41% of those who received the invitation). Of these 148 mothers, 108 had a child who was between the ages of

3 and 18 and who was living with them at least half of the time. This restriction on age of child was made because the measure of children's social competence has been validated for children between 3 and 18 (Ellsworth, 1979; Pett, 1979). Although 41% is a low response rate and requires additional information to help evaluate the representativeness of the sample, the rate is comparable to other published research on divorce, as noted by Furstenberg and Spanier (1984).

Sample characteristics. Although court records were used to identify the sample, most of the respondents were Caucasian. An analysis of the 1986 court records indicated that only 10 blacks (5 couples) had filed for divorce in the county. About 42% of the mothers stopped their formal education after high school, 38% completed non-college training or some college, and 20% completed college. Seventy-nine percent were currently employed and the median number of hours worked per week was 40. The modal occupation status was clerical and sales. Current median net monthly income was $915 (range 0-$5,000), and most of the mothers defined their economic situation as "struggling" (37%) or "doing okay" (45%).

The mean age for mothers was 32 (range 21-45; SD = 5.3). The median length of marriage was 10 years (SD = 5.2) and the median length of separation was 6 months (SD = 10.5). About 85% had either one or two children. The target children in multiple-child families were selected randomly so that mother's responses were unique to a particular child.

Two different procedures were used to evaluate the representativeness of this sample. The first procedure was to compare empirically the survey respondents and nonrespondents using the background data available from court records. Responding and nonresponding mothers were compared on the following variables: age, education, occupational status, income, employment status, length of marriage, and number of children. There were no group differences on level of education, occupational status, income, and number of children. Group differences existed for age, length of marriage, and employment status. Nonresponding mothers were older (t (139) = −3.48, p < .01), had been married longer (t (135) = −5.15, p = .04) and were more likely to be employed ($X^2 = 4.28, p = .04$) than the responding mothers.

The second procedure used to assess sample representativeness was to compare the sample survey data with data from the 1986 Census (U.S. Bureau of the Census, 1987). Using nonstatistical visual inspection, the sample of mothers used for this study seemed to be a little more educated and to have higher employment rates than the U.S. average of divorced mothers. The groups seemed comparable on age and income. Thus, the comparison between respondents and nonrespondents coupled with the examination of relevant census data indicated that this sample of responding mothers was fairly representative of the Caucasian divorcing population (with the exception of a slight bias in education).

Measures

Dependent variables. Children's social competence (CSC) was measured by a revised version of the Child and Adolescent Profile (CAAP) scale (Ellsworth, 1979; Pett, 1979, 1982). The CAAP was chosen because it has been validated for children between the ages of 3 and 18 and because it includes measures of both anti and prosocial dimensions of CSC. Mothers were asked to rate specific child behaviors during the past month using a 1 (never) to 4 (often) response scale. Based on a factor analysis of responses from mothers in this study, the following subscales were developed by averaging individual subscale items: dependency, aggression, anxiety/withdrawal, and productivity. Alpha coefficients for the scales were .86 for dependency, .84 for aggression, .82 for anxiety/withdrawal, and .80 for productivity (see Table 1).

Parenting variables. Four indicators of mother's parenting were used. *Loss of time spent with child* since the separation was measured by the statement, "I have had less time to spend with my children." Responses were dichotomized as yes (coded 1 for the dummy; n = 59) or no (coded 0 for the dummy; n = 49). *Companionship* was measured by the following question: "How often do you and your child have a good time together?" (Berg & Kurdek, 1983). The scale ranged from 1 (never) to 5 (always). *Coercion* was measured as the sum of mother's self-reported control behaviors used frequently in the past week, including yelling, threatening, hitting or spanking their child. Evidence of content validity for this measure of coercion can be found in Dadds (1987) who states that yelling and threatening are the most common forms of parental aggressive behavior toward children. Cronbach's alpha is not an appropriate indicator of reliability for this composite because aggregation rather than covariation is the relevant characteristic measured. *Daily involvement* was measured using Ahrons' (1983) parental involvement scale. Mothers were asked to record the amount of involvement with their child in 11 activities such as running errands, discipline, dress and grooming, planning and preparing meals. The scale ranged from 1 (not at all) to 5 (very much) and Cronbach's alpha was .88. Mother's reports of the *frequency of paternal visitation* was measured by asking, "How often does the nonresidential parent see the child?" Responses of the seven-point scale ranged from never (1) to daily (7).

Moderating variables. The three variables hypothesized to moderate the relationship between mothers' parenting and CSC postseparation were child's *sex, age,* and *family economic hardship.* Of the 107 cases studied, 51 included girls (coded 0 in the sex dummy variable) and 57 included boys (coded 1 in the sex dummy); 40 included pre-schoolers (coded 0 in the age dummy #1), 42 children ages 6 to 11 (coded 1 in age dummies #1 and #2), and 26 adolescents (coded 0 in the age dummy #2). There were 40 mothers who reported they were struggling economically (coded 1 in the dummy) and 67 who reported that they were "doing okay" or better (coded 0 in the dummy).

Control variables. Time from separation was measured in months. Maternal education was measured by an eight-point ordinal scale that ranged from "grade school or less" (1) to "graduate degree" (8). *Parental conflict* was measured using 16 items from Berg and Kurdek's Separation Inventory (1983) that address parenting-related disagreements. Ahrons (1983) has provided evidence of construct validity for this scale and inter-item consistency reliability for the present sample was .93. Mother's *psychosocial well-being* was measured using an averaged composite of four measures: self-esteem (Rosenberg, 1965), emotional affect (Bradburn & Caplovitz, 1965), psychosomatic symptomatology (Spanier & Thomp-

186

Table 1

Means, Standard Deviations, Alphas, and Correlations of Variables

Variables	(1)	(2)	(3)	(4)	(5)	(6)	(7)	(8)	(9)	(10)	(11)	(12)	(13)
Dependent													
1) aggression	1.00	.36	.48	-.27	.13	-.15	-.26	.24	.11	.11	-.02	.01	-.16
2) dependency		1.00	.38	-.31	.11	-.05	-.16	.30	.08	.06	-.03	.09	-.10
3) anxiety			1.00	-.23	.11	-.08	-.26	.19	.06	.00	.00	.07	-.30
4) productivity				1.00	-.09	.21	.16	-.30	-.07	.13	-.04	.02	.32
Independent													
5) less time					1.00	-.04	-.19	.01	.03	.03	.07	.02	-.22
6) daily involvement						1.00	.31	-.07	.10	.16	.00	.11	.12
7) companionship							1.00	-.13	-.02	.25	.03	.11	.29
8) coercion								1.00	-.07	.02	.10	.01	-.12
9) father visitation									1.00	.08	-.23	.22	.03

Control

										10	11	12	13
10) mother education										1.00	-.21	-.05	-.06
11) separation months											1.00	-.32	.02
12) coparental conflict												1.00	-.02
13) mother psychosocial well-being													1.00
Mean	2.04	2.53	2.07	3.12	.55	4.53	4.13	1.23	4.41	4.30	9.32	1.92	3.38
Standard Deviation	.78	.75	.63	.61	.50	.53	.64	1.05	1.65	1.59	10.48	.72	.68
Alpha	.84	.86	.82	.80	---	.88	---	---	---	---	.93	---	---

Note: Analyses are based on 108 mothers. Correlations above .18 are significant at $p < .05$.

son, 1984), and life satisfaction (Spanier & Thompson, 1984). Validity evidence of these measures can be found in Buehler (1989). Mother's age was not included as a control variable because it correlated .07 with child's age.

Analytic Procedures

The hypotheses were tested using a hierarchial multiple regression technique that included interaction terms to test for significant moderating effects. Thus, for each measure of CSC there were four regression equations calculated: one that included the direct and moderating effects of child sex, two that included the direct and moderating effects of child age (two different dummy variables), and one that included the direct and moderating effects of family economic hardship. To avoid potential statistical problems associated with the use of interaction terms in multiple regression analyses, the moderator variables were centered using the mean before interaction terms were created (James & Brett, 1984; Smith & Sasaki, 1979.)

The probability criterion used in the analysis of direct effects was $p < .05$ and of interaction effects was $p < .07$ (because the tests for interactions were exploratory). Significant interaction terms should be interpreted as partial terms, i.e., the term is significant controlling for the parenting variables, the control variables, and the other four interaction terms. For each analytic equation, the regression assumptions were assessed by examining the residual plots for each dependent variable. The normality, linearity, and constant variance assumptions seemed valid for each equation.

RESULTS

Most importantly, with a few exceptions that will be discussed, sex of child, age of child, and family economic hardship *did not moderate* the relationship between various parenting variables and CSC postseparation. Of 20 possible interaction terms based on sex of child (five parenting variables times four dependent variables), only two were significant and both related to maternal coercion.

First, the relationship between coercion and child dependency differed for sons and daughters (Beta = .24, p = .02). The relationship was positive for both groups (more coercion related to more dependency and vice versa), but the relationship was stronger for sons than daughters. Thus, mother's coercive control attempts affected son's dependency behaviors more than daughter's. Second, the relationship between coercion and child productivity also differed for sons and daughters (Beta = −.23, p = .02). The relationship was negative for both groups, but, again, the relationship was stronger for sons than daughters. Both of these interactions were in the hypothesized direction, but it is important to place them in context. Only one parenting variable out of five, coercion, and only two aspects of CSC out of four, dependency and productivity, resulted in differential patterns for sons and daughters.

In comparing children ages 6 through 11 with preschoolers, again only 2 of 20 interaction terms were significant. The relationship between loss of time with mother and child aggression differed for school-aged children and preschoolers (Beta = .21, p = .06). There was almost no correlation between the two for preschoolers, but the association was strong for school aged children. A loss in time with mother since the separation was associated with much higher levels of child aggression. The relationship between mother's daily involvement and aggression also differed for the two age groups (Beta = −.21, p = .07), and evidenced the same patterns as loss of time. Although limited in scope, direction of these patterns supported the hypothesis that the effects of parenting on CSC are stronger for school-aged children than preschoolers.

In comparing children ages 6 through 11 with adolescents, two of the interaction terms were significant. First, the relationship between mother's coercion and anxiety/withdrawal differed for the two age groups (Beta = −.26, p = .05). The relationship was positive for adolescents and negative for school-aged children. This pattern did not support the hypothesis. Second, the relationship between having less time with mother and child aggression was much stronger for school-aged children than it was for adolescents (Beta = .35, p = .01). This effect was hypothesized.

Finally, only one interaction term was significant when family economic hardship was the moderating variable. As hypothesized, the negative relationship between companionship with mother and child anxiety was much stronger in families who were struggling financially than in those families who had adequate finances (Beta = -31, $p = .002$).

As would be expected based on the zero-order correlations, controlling for mother's education, time from separation, and coparental conflict did not change any of these results. Although mother's psychosocial well-being was related to her reports of child anxiety and productivity, controlling for this shared variance did not change the patterns of statistical interaction.

In sum, these results indicated that generally the effects of mother's parenting and father's visitation on CSC postseparation were rather uniform, unaffected by variation in child sex, age, and family economic hardship. The few significant interactions were in hypothesized directions, with the exception of comparisons between school-aged children and adolescents. Focusing on the direct effects of the parenting variables, maternal coercion was the strongest variable of the five. It was related to higher levels of child aggression, dependency, anxiety/withdrawal, and to lower levels of productivity.

IMPLICATIONS FOR PRACTITIONERS

Some of the findings from this study replicated those from past research by confirming that mother's coercive control attempts are associated with higher levels of antisocial behavior problems in children. To a more limited extent, a positive, warm relationship with mother also predicted higher levels of children's social competence. With a few exceptions, these findings described children/ youth of both sexes between ages 3 and 18 in families of varying levels of financial adequacy. The exceptions indicated two patterns: (a) when compared with daughters, some externalized aspects of son's social competence (i.e., dependency and productivity) were affected more strongly by mother's coercive control attempts, and (b) school-aged children were upset by the reduced time spent with their mothers since the separation. This upsettedness manifested primarily in aggressive behavior.

Before discussing the implications of these findings, it is important to recognize and evaluate the limitations of this research. Although the sample seems fairly representative of the U. S. Caucasian, recently separated population and there were few differences between respondents and nonrespondents on biographical data, the findings must be interpreted cautiously until replicated using a national sample. A second major concern stems from the sole use of mother reports to obtain the data. The validity threat created by this method of data collection is that the obtained correlation between the independent and dependent variable may be due to shared agent variance as well as true systematic variance. As noted in the literature review, researchers have found that mother's reports of child outcomes are overly influenced by their own well-being. Thus, in this study, mother's psychosocial well-being was used as a control variable to help reduce the inflating effects of systematic error variance. Although it is certain that this control did not entirely solve the problems created by shared agent variance, the effects were reduced.

There are at least two major implications of these findings for practitioners. Most importantly, practitioners need a thorough understanding of the definition and interpretation of statistical interaction terms. They need to understand how these effects differ from direct effects, and to learn how to sort through evidence supporting one or the other. Without this understanding, it is difficult to identify generalizations or profiles about potential client vulnerabilities in various contexts. For example, most practitioners are aware of the research suggesting that sons exhibit more aggressive behaviors postseparation than do daughters. Most also are aware that mothers who use a characteristically coercive parenting style are more likely to have overly aggressive children than mothers who use other parenting styles. However, given the current state of research knowledge, it would be inaccurate to conclude that the effects of maternal coercion on child aggression are stronger for sons than for daughters. This sex interaction was not found in this study and has not been found in other studies (e.g., Dodge, Bates, & Pettit, 1990), with the possible exception of Hetherington's work. Thus, an understanding of the differences between direct and interactive effects will enhance the practitioner's ability to make wise choices concerning intervention goals and potential areas of client vulnerability.

The second implication of this study focuses on specific content that needs to be included in programs for divorcing parents or in therapeutic work with divorcing clients. The findings from this study suggest that mother's control/discipline behaviors need to be addressed regardless of child sex, age, and family economic well-being. In addition, however, these findings also indicate that mother's who have sons are particularly vulnerable and may require extra attention in terms of parent education. Improving/maintaining the companionate aspects of the mother-child relationship also is important to include as an intervention goal for all parents, regardless of child sex or age.

Finally, these findings suggest tentatively that children ages 6 to 11 have a difficult time adjusting to spending less time with their mothers postseparation. (This loss of time resulted primarily from increased employment activity.) Thus, it seems important to have children talk about their feelings with regards to this loss. Also, it would be helpful to develop a few easy, "special" activities that mother's can incorporate into their schedules that may help counteract their increased time away from home. Although doing these activities occasionally may not take extra time or be costly, their conception and planning take attention and foresight. Practitioners can help families cope with some the changes brought on by the marital separation by facilitating this process of conceptualizing and planning.

REFERENCES

Ahrons, C. (1983). Predictors of paternal involvement post-divorce: Mothers' and fathers' perceptions. *Journal of Divorce, 6,* 55-69.

Allison, P. D., & Furstenberg, F. (1989). How marital dissolution affects children: Variations by age and sex. *Developmental Psychology, 25,* 540-549.

Ambert, A. (1984). Children's behavior to custodial parents. *Journal of Marriage and the Family, 46,* 443-461.

Belsky, J. (1990). Parental and nonparental child care and children's socioemotional development: A decade in review. *Journal of Marriage and the Family, 52,* 885-903.

Berg, B. & Kurdek, L. (1983). Parent separation inventory. Unpublished survey.

Block, J. H., Block, J., & Gjerde, P. (1986). The personality of children prior to divorce: A prospective study. *Child Development, 57,* 827-840.

Bradburn, N. M., & Caplovitz, D, (1965). *Reports on happiness.* Chicago: University of Chicago Press.

Brody, G., & Forehand, R. (1988). Multiple determinants of parenting: Research findings and implications for the divorce process. In E. M. Hetherington & J. D. Arasteh (Eds.), *Impact of divorce, single-parenting, and stepparenting on children* (pp. 117 -133). Hillsdale, NJ: Erlbaum.

Buehler, C. (1989). The influence of employment and economic factors on mothers' psychosocial well-being and children's social competence following marital separation. *Family Perspective, 23,* 165-183.

Camara, K. A., & Resnick, G. (1988). Interparental conflict and cooperation: Factors moderating children's postdivorce adjustment. In E. M. Hetherington & J. D. Arasteh (Eds.), *Impact of divorce, single-parenting and stepparenting on children* (pp. 169- 195). Hillsdale, NJ: Erlbaum.

Colletta, N. (1983). Stressful lives: The situation of divorced mothers and their children. *Journal of Divorce, 6,* 19-31.

Dadds, M. R. (1987). Families and the origins of child behavior problems. *Family Process, 26,* 341-357.

Demo, D. H., & Acock, A. C. (1988). The impact of divorce on children. *Journal of Marriage and the Family, 50,* 619-648.

Dodge, K. A., Bates, J. E., Pettit, G. S. (1990). Mechanisms in the cycle of violence. *Science, 250,* 1678-1683.

Ellsworth, R. (1979). CAAP Scale: The measurement of child and adolescent adjustment. Roanoke: Institute for Program Evaluation.

Emery, R. E. (1982). Interpersonal conflict and the children of discord and divorce. *Psychological Bulletin, 2,* 310-330.

Emery, R. E., Hetherington, E. M., & DiLalla, L. F. (1983). In H. W. Stevenson & A. W. Siegel (Eds.), *Divorce, Children, and Social Policy* (pp. 189-266). Chicago: University of Chicago Press.

Erikson, E. (1968). *Identity: Youth and crisis.* NY: Norton.

Forgatch, M. S., Patterson, G. R., & Skinner, M. L. (1988). A mediational model for the effect of divorce on antisocial behavior in boys. In E. M. Hetherington & J. D. Arasteh (Eds.), *Impact of divorce single-parenting and stepparenting on children* (pp. 135-154). Hillsdale, NJ: Erlbaum.

Furstenberg, F., & Nord, C. (1985). Parenting apart: Patterns of childrearing after marital disruption and parental contact. *American Sociological Review, 48,* 656- 668.

Furstenberg, F. F. & Seltzer, J. A. (1986). Divorce and child development. In P. Adler & P. Adler (Eds.), *Sociological Studies of Child Development,* (Vol. 3, pp. 137-160). Greenwich, CT: JAI Press.

Furstenberg, F., & Spanier, G. (1984). *Recycling the family: Remarriage after divorce.* Beverly Hills, CA: Sage Publications, Inc.

Glick, P. (1984). Marriage, divorce, and living arrangements: Prospective changes. *Journal of Family Issues, 5,* 7-26.

Guidubaldi, J., & Perry, J. D. (1984). Divorce, socioeconomic status and children's cognitive-social competence at school entry. *American Journal of Orthopsychiatry, 54*, 459-468.

Guidubaldi, J., & Perry, J. D. (1985). Divorce and mental health sequelae for children: A two year follow-up of a nationwide sample. *Journal of the American Academy of Child Psychiatry, 24*, 531-537.

Guidubaldi, J., Cleminshaw, H., Perry, J., & Kehle, T. (1983, March). The impact of parental divorce on children: A report of the nationwide NASP study. Paper presented at the annual convention of the National Association of School Psychologists, Detroit, MI.

Hetherington, E. M. (1987). Family relations six years after divorce. In K. Pasley, & M. Ihinger-Tallman (Eds.), *Remarriage and stepparenting: Current research and theory* (pp. 185-205). NY: Guilford.

Hetherington, E. M. (1989). Coping with family transitions: Winners, losers, and survivors. *Child Development, 60*, 1-14.

Hetherington, E. M., & Camara, K. A. (1984). Families in transition: The process of dissolution and reconstitution. In R. Parke (Ed.), *Review of child development research* (Vol. 3, pp. 398-439). Chicago: University of Chicago press.

Hetherington, E. M., Cox, M., & Cox, R. (1982). Effects of divorce on parents and children. In M. Lamb (Ed.), *Nontraditional families* (pp. 233-288). Hillsdale, NJ: Erlbaum.

Jacobson, D. S. (1978). The impact of marital separation/divorce on children: III. Parent-child communication and child adjustment, and regression analysis of findings from overall study. *Journal of Divorce, 2*, 175-194.

James, L. R., & Brett, J. M. (1984). Mediators, moderators, and tests for mediation. *Journal of Applied Psychology, 69*, 307-321.

Kalter, N., & Rembar, J. (1981). The significance of a child's age at the time of parental divorce. *American Journal of Orthopsychiatry, 51*, 85-100.

Kurdek, L. A. (1987). Children's adjustment to divorce: An ecological perspective. In J. P. Vincent (Ed.), *Advances in family intervention, assessment, and theory* (Vol. 4; pp. 1- 31). Greenwich, CT: JAI Press.

Kurdek, L. A., & Berg, B. (1983). Correlates of children's adjustment to their parents' divorce. In L. A. Kurdek (Ed.), *Children and divorce* (pp. 47-60). San Francisco: Jossey-Bass Inc., Publishers.

Patterson, G. R., DeBaryshe, B. D., Ramsey, E. (1989). A developmental perspective on antisocial behavior. *American Psychologist, 44*, 329-335.

Pett, M. (1982). Correlates of children's social adjustment following divorce. *Journal of Divorce, 5*(4), 25-39.

Pett, M. (1979). Predictors of postdivorce adjustment in single-parent families. Unpublished doctoral dissertation. University of Utah.

Peterson, J. L., & Zill, N. (1986). Marital disruption, parent-child relationships, and behavior problems in children. *Journal of Marriage and the Family, 48*, 295-307.

Rosenberg, N. (1965). *Society and the adolescent self-image*. Princeton, NJ: Princeton University Press.

Shaw, D. S., & Emery, R. E. (1988). Chronic family adversity and school-age children's adjustment. *Journal of American Academy of Child and Adolescent Psychiatry, 27*, 200-206.

Smith, K. W. & Sasaki, M. S. (1979). Decreasing multicollinearity: A method for models with multiplicative functions. *Sociological Methods and Research, 8*, 35-56.

Spanier, G., & Thompson, L. (1984). *Parting: The aftermath of separation and divorce.* Newbury Park, CA: Sage Publications Inc.

Tschann, J. M., Johnston, J. R., Kline, M., & Wallerstein, J. S. (1989). Family process and children's functioning during divorce. *Journal of Marriage and the Family, 51*, 431-444.

Tschann, J. M., Johnston, J. R., Kline, M., & Wallerstein, J. S. (1990). Conflict, loss, change and parent-child relationships: Predicting children's adjustment during divorce. *Journal of Divorce, 13*, 1-22.

U.S. Bureau of the Census. (1987). Household and family characteristics: March 1986. (Current Population Reports, Series P-20). Washington, DC: U.S. Government Printing Office.

Wallerstein, J. S., Corbin, S. B., & Lewis, J. M. (1988). Children of divorce: A ten year study. In E. M. Hetherington & J. D. Arasteh (Eds.), *Impact of divorce, single-parenting and stepparenting on children* (pp. 198-214). Hillsdale, NJ: Erlbaum.

Zaslow, M. J. (1987, September). Sex differences in children's response to parental divorce. Paper presented at the Symposium on Sex Differences in Children's Responses to Psychosocial Stress, Woods Hole, MA.

Implications of Divorce on Reasons for Living in Older Adolescents

Jon B. Ellis
C. Denise Russell

SUMMARY. To assess any possible differences in reasons for living between adolescents from divorced families and those from "intact" families, 286 older adolescent age undergraduates were, administered the Reasons for Living Inventory (RFL). Adolescents from divorced families revealed lower Responsibility to Family beliefs, but other adaptive cognitive characteristics were not different. Various demographics were shown to have some impact on reasons for living, especially the age of the child at the time of the divorce.

Divorce has been shown to increase the chances of negative effects on the psychological health of family members. Research has consistently demonstrated these effects on families with children (Bloom, Asher, & White, 1978; Emery, 1982; Guidubaldi, Perry, Cleminshaw, & McLoughlin, 1983; Hetherington, 1979, Kurdels, 1981; Wallerstein,1984). Children may even experience more problems in divorced families than ill families where a parent has died (Douglas, Ross, Hammond, & Mulligan, 1986). It has been shown that while younger children may experience more problems following a divorce, adolescents and older children may experience more problems later on (Hetherington, Cox, & Cox, 1978; Wallerstein, 1984). Thus, there appears to be sufficient interest and rationale to examine how divorce may have affected some of the adaptive characteristics which adolescents typically display.

Jon B. Ellis, PhD, is Assistant Professor in the Department of Psychology at East Tennessee State University, Johnson City, TN 37614-0002.
C. Denise Russell, MA, was a graduate student in that department.

© 1992 by The Haworth Press, Inc. All rights reserved.

197

Over 60 percent of couples seeking a divorce have children still living within the home (Blades, Gosse, McKay & Rogers, 1984). Wallerstein (1988) presents divorce as a continuum of changing family relationships which begins during the failing years of the marriage and extends over many years. For children, divorce usually occurs during the formative years of development. It is during these formative years that most individuals are forming their beliefs about life. The disruption of the family through divorce may cause children to assume new roles, beliefs, and expectations about their lives.

After a divorce a child's responsibility to family is affected by the loss of one parent within the home. The child is often responsible for the care of younger children and assumes more household chores (Blades, Gosse, McKay & Rogers, 1984). In some cases one parent may become the victim of the divorce and attempt to put the child in a supportive role, thereby creating role reversal between parent and child (Little, 1982). Coping beliefs are utilized during the divorce and the years following in order to survive the breakup of the family. If parental support is inadequate during this time, these beliefs and skills may be developed deficiently, causing stress later in life when these skills are needed and absent. Wallerstein (1988) found that children tended to do well if mothers and fathers resumed parenting roles and allowed a continuing relationship with both parents.

A divorce may cause a child to feel a sense of abandonment. The possibility of strengthened commitments to their own children may produce higher beliefs from individuals of divorced families. Wallerstein (1988) views the families of these children as being more vulnerable which could result in less child-related beliefs.

There may also be implications in the development of social and moral beliefs. The beliefs formed by a child in regards to the divorce may be directly related to their understanding of the divorce. If a child is given definite information as to the reasons for the divorce they are less likely to make up their own answers (Blade et al., 1984). If the child feels the divorce was morally wrong (mom or dad was bad) or socially unacceptable (comments by others) then these beliefs may be affected.

The effects of divorce can create situational factors which may contribute to maladaptive psychological development. One area which has received little attention is the relationship between divorce and suicidal behavior of children from divorced families.

Suicidal individuals have been described as having problems with two major aspects of living: affect and cognition. In terms of affect, they have been described as depressed (e.g., Birtchnell, 1981; Evenson, 1983), excitable (Sonneck, Grunberger, & Ringel, 1976), and highly arousable (Mehrabian & Weinstein, 1985). In terms of cognition, they have been described as rigid (Neuringer, 1964; Patsiokas, Clum, & Luscomb, 1979), particularly under stress (Schotte & Clum, 1982), impulsive (Bhagat, 1976; Cantor, 1976), ambivalent toward life and death (Orbach, Fesbach, Carlson, Glaubman, & Gross, 1983), hopeless (Beck, 1963; Beck, Steer, Kovacs, & Garrison, 1985), and as having a low social desirability response set (Linehan & Nielsen, 1981).

Nearly all of the research in both areas has focused on negative aspects of these characteristics. Focusing on adaptive, life-maintaining characteristics which may keep a person from considering suicide has received little attention, despite the fact that there are sound theoretical and clinical reasons for doing so. From a clinical perspective, testimonials have indicated that beliefs about life, and expectations for the future, are instrumental in keeping many people alive through extreme stress.

In an attempt to correct this deficiency, Linehan, Goodstein, Nielsen, and Chiles (1983) developed the Reasons for Living Inventory (RFL), a scale having as its purpose the identification of beliefs that are potentially important reasons for not committing suicide. It requires a rating of how important each reason would be for living, if suicide were being considered.

METHOD

Subjects

Subjects were 286 older adolescent aged undergraduates (168 women; 118 men) from a southern university. They ranged in age from 17 to 25 years (*M* = 19.5, sd 1.8). Everyone completed a

demographic questionnaire which included whether or not they
were from a "divorced" family and, if so, at what age a parent left
the home.

One hundred and ninety students (66. 9%) were reared in "intact" families in which the parents were not divorced. Seventy
seven (27. 1%) reported that their parents were divorced. The age of
the student at the time of his/her parents' divorce ranged from less
than one year to 22 years with a mean of 9.9 years.

Instruments

The Expanded Reasons for Living Inventory (RFL; Linehan,
Goodstein, Nielsen, & Chiles, 1983) is a 72-item inventory which
measures beliefs and expectancies that are reasons for not committing suicide should it be considered. Each statement is rated on a
scale of 1 ("not at all important"), to 6 ("extremely important").
Factor analysis indicated six subscales: Survival and Coping Beliefs, Responsibility to Family, Child Concerns, Fear of Suicide,
Fear of Social Disapproval, and Moral Objections. Another subscale, Responsibility to Friends, was deleted by the authors after
four factor analyses, but has been recommended by M. M. Linehan
because they seem to tap a separate factor, responsibility to friends,
which may also be a reason for not committing suicide (personal
communication, October 2, 1986). In terms of reliability, the RFL
has been shown to be moderately strong, with Chronbach alphas on
each subscale ranging from .72 to .89 (Linehan et al., 1983; Range &
Steede, 1988). Ill terms of validity, the RFL differentiates between
suicidal and nonsuicidal individuals in both inpatient and outpatient
settings (Linehan et al., 1983).

RESULTS

A 2(Divorced vs. Intact) $\times$ 2(Gender) analysis of variance
(ANOVA) was utilized to examine differences between groups on
the PFL subscales and total score. As expected, adolescents from
intact families reported higher scores on the Responsibility to Family

subscale, F(1,251 = 6.71 p < .01. Women scored higher than did men on the Fear of Suicide subscale, F(1,251 = 5.01, p < 05. The difference between men's and women's scores also approached significance on the Responsibility to Family and the Child Related Concerns subscales. On both scales, women's scores were higher. No significant interaction effects were revealed (Table 1).

A Multiple Repression analysis was also utilized to examine any effect which various demographic variables might have on RFL scores. These variables included subject's age, age at parent's divorce, gender, presence of a caretaker such as a boyfriend, girlfriend, aunt, uncle, etc., stepparent, visits by parent who left home, parent working outside of home, birth order and sibling.

Age at the time of divorce accounted for a significant amount of variance between the two groups on the total RFL score, Survival and Coping Beliefs, Responsibility to Family, Fear of Social Disapproval, and Responsibility to Friends subscales. The presence of a stepparent in the home also had a significant effect on Survival and Coping Beliefs.

DISCUSSION

As might be expected, older adolescents who were reared in homes with divorced parents reveal less responsibility to family beliefs. Based on the results of this study, these beliefs are not changed with the presence of a stepparent, other family support, or other apparent variables related to the healthy adjustment of a child in a divorced home.

One variable which does appear to make a difference concerns the age of a child at the time of her/his parents divorce. This partially replicates past research which has indicated that the younger the child, the better prognosis for healthy psychological development. These results suggest that the cognitive characteristics which may keep people from committing suicide (reasons for living) are stronger among people who were younger at the time of the divorce.

An encouraging aspect of this study involves the lack of differences between the two groups of adolescents. Although their scores on these very important adaptive characteristics are not significant-

Table 1

RFL Means and Standard Deviations for All Subjects

Survival and Coping Beliefs

    Divorced   (n=77)   5.08 (.81)

    Intact   (n=190)   5.05 (.77)

    All   (n=286)   5.08 (.76)

Responsibility to Family

    Divorced   4.48 (1.19)

    Intact   4.84 (.95)*

    All   4.72 (1.03)

Child Related Concerns

    Divorced   4.15 (1.80)

    Intact   4.33 (1.72)

    All   4.25 (1.75)

Fear of Suicide

    Divorced   3.04 (1.18)

    Intact   3.00 (1.17)

    All   2.96 (1.18)

Fear of Social Disapproval

    Divorced   3.07 (1.57)

    Intact   3.19 (1.55)

    All   3.13 (1.56)

Table 1 continued

Moral Objections

Divorced	4.23 (1.47)
Intact	4.45 (1.34)
All	4.34 (1.40)

Responsibility to Friends

Divorced	4.07 (.91)
Intact	4.21 (.83)
All	4.17 (.85)

Total RFL Score

Divorced	4.31 (.77)
Intact	4.37 (.73)
All	4.35 (.74)

Note: Items ranged from 1 (low) to 6 (high).

*p<.01

ly different from other adolescents, their mean score was slightly higher (5.08 vs. 5.05).

This study also further shows the relevance of the Reasons for Living Inventory. Not only is the RFL potentially useful clinically, but it also has strong research possibilities. Indeed, it has several advantages over other research instruments. First, its positive focus (on reasons for *not* committing suicide) is much less noxious than the negative focus of other instruments. One would certainly want to avoid any suicide assessment instrument that induced suicidal thinking. The RFL sidesteps this criticism by focusing on reasons *not* to commit suicide. Second, the RFL's six subscales are an advantage over most other research instruments in the area. These different aspects of the RFL can provide much more information than would be available from a total score alone.

REFERENCES

Beck, A. (1963). Thinking and depression: Idiosyncratic content and cognitive distortion. *Archives of General Psychiatry 9*, 324-333.

Beck, A. Steer, R., Kovacs, M., & Garrison B. (1985). Hopelessness and eventual suicide: A 10-year prospective study of patients hospitalized with suicidal ideation. *American Journal of Psychiatry, 142*, 559-563.

Bhagat, M. (1976). The spouses of attempted suicides: A personality Study. *British Journal of Psychiatry, 128*, 44-46.

Birtchnell, J. (1961). Some familial and clinical characteristics of female suicidal psychiatric patients. *British Journal of Psychiatry, 138*, 381-390.

Blades, J., Gosse,R., McKay, M. & Rogers, P. (1984). *The divorce book*. Oakland, CA: New Harbinger Publications.

Bloom, B. Asher, S. , & White S. (1978). Marital disruption as a stressor: A review and analysis. *Psychological Bulletin*, 85, 867-894.

Cantor, P. (1976). Personality characteristics found among youthful female suicide attempters. *Journal of Abnormal Psychology, 85*, 324-329.

Douglas, J., Ross, T., Hammond, W., & Mulligan, D. (1986). Delinquency and social class. *British Journal of Criminology, 6*, 294-302.

Emery, R. (1982). Interparental conflict and the children of discord and divorce. *Psychological Bulletin, 92*, 310-330.

Evenson, R. (1983). Community adjustment of patients who threaten and attempt suicide. *Psychological Reports, 52*, 127-132.

Guidubaldi, J., Perry, J., Cleminshaw, H. & McLoughlin, C. (1983). The impact of parental divorce on children: Report of the nationwide NASP study. *School Psychology Review, 12*, 300-323.

Heath, P., & MacKinnon, C. (1988). Factors related to the social competence of children in single-parent families. *Journal of Divorce, 11*, 49-66.

Hetherington, E. (1979). Divorce: A child's perspective. *American Psychologist, 34*, 851-858.

Hetherington, E., Cox M., & Cox, R. (1978). The aftermath of divorce. In J. H. Stevens & M. Mathews (Eds.), *Mother/child and father/child relationships*. Washington DC: National Association of Education of Children.

Kurdek, L. , (1988). Social support of divorced single mothers and their children. *Journal of Divorce, 11*, 166-188.

Kurdek, L. (1981). An integrative perspective on children's divorce adjustment. *American Psychologist, 36*, 856-866.

Linehan, M., Goodstein, J., Nielson, S. & Chiles, J. (1983). Reasons for staying alive when you are thinking of killing yourself: The Reasons for Living Inventory. *Journal of Consulting and Clinical Psychology, 51*, 276-286.

Linehan, M., & Nielsen, S. (1981). Assessment of suicide ideation and parasuicide: Hopelessness and social desirability. *Journal of Consulting and Clinical Psychology, 49*, 773-775.

Little, M. (1982). *Family breakup*. San Francisco: Jossey-Bass Inc.

Mehrabian, A , & Weinstein, L. (1985). Temperament characteristics of suicide attempters. *Journal of Consulting and Clinical Psychology, 53,* 544-546.

Neuringer, C. (1964). Rigid thinking in suicidal individuals. *Journal of Consulting Psychology, 28,* 54-58.

Orbach, I., Fesbach, S., Carlson, G., Glaubman, H., & Gross, Y. (1983). Attraction and repulsion by life and death in suicidal and normal children. *Journal of Consulting and Clinical Psychology, 51,* 661-670.

Patsiokas, A., Clum, B., & Luscomb, R. (1979). Cognitive characteristics of suicide attempters. *Journal of Consulting and Clinical Psychology, 47,* 478-484.

Schotte, D. , & Clum, G. (1982). Suicide ideation in a college population: A test of a model. *Journal of Consulting and Clinical Psychology, 50,* 690-696.

Soneck, G. Grunbeerger, J., & Ringel,E. (1976). Experimental contribution to evaluation of the suicidal risk of depressive patients. *Psychiatrica Clinica, 9* 84-96.

Suicide among youth. (Fall, 1987). Update from U. S. Department of Health and Human Services.

Wallerstein, J. (1984). Children of divorce: Preliminary report of a 10-year-follow-up of young children. *American Journal of Orthopsychiatry, 54,* 444-458.

Wallerstein, J. (1988). Children after divorce: Wounds that don't heal. *Perspectives in Psychiatric Care, 34,* 107-113.